WORKING WITH BILINGUAL
LANGUAGE DISABILITY

Therapy In Practice
Series Editor: Jo Campling

This series of books is aimed at 'therapists' concerned with rehabilitation in a very broad sense. The intended audience particularly includes occupational therapists, physiotherapists and speech therapists, but many titles will also be of interest to nurses, psychologists, medical staff, social workers, teachers or volunteer workers. Some volumes will be interdisciplinary, others aimed at one particular profession. All titles will be comprehensive but concise, and practical but with due reference to relevant theory and evidence. They are not research monographs but focus on professional practice, and will be of value to both students and qualified personnel.

Titles Available

Occupational Therapy for Children with Disabilities
Dorothy E. Penso

Living Skills for Mentally Handicapped People
Christine Peck and Chia Swee Hong

Rehabilitation of the Older Patient
Edited by Amanda J. Squires

Physiotherapy and the Elderly Patient
Paul Wagstaff and Davis Coakley

Rehabilitation of the Severely Brain-Injured Adult
Edited by Ian Fussey and Gordon Muir Giles

Communication Problems in Elderly People
Rosemary Gravell

Occupational Therapy Practice in Psychiatry
Linda Finlay

Counselling Skills for Health Professionals
Philip Burnard

Titles in Preparation

Modern Electrotherapy
Mary Dyson and Christopher Hayne

Movement Exercises for Language Difficulties
M. Nash-Wortham

Management in Occupational Therapy
Zielfa B. Maslin

Community Occupational Therapy with Mentally Handicapped People
Debbie Isaac

Understanding Dysphasia
Lesley Jordan and Rita Twiston Davies

Dysarthria: Theory and Therapy
Sandra J. Robertson

Occupational Therapy for the Brain-Injured Adult
Jo Clark-Wilson and Gordon Muir Giles

Speech and Language Problems in Children
Dilys A. Treharne

Acute Head Injury: Practical Management in Rehabilitation
Ruth Garner

Occupational Therapy in Stroke Rehabilitation
Simon Thompson and Maryanne Morgan

Physiotherapy in Respiratory and Intensive Care
Alexandra Hough

Working with Bilingual Language Disability

Edited by
DEIRDRE M. DUNCAN

London New York
CHAPMAN AND HALL

First published in 1989 by Chapman and Hall Ltd
11 New Fetter Lane, London EC4P 4EE
Published in the USA by Routledge, Chapman and Hall
29 West 35th Street, New York NY 10001

© 1989 Deirdre M. Duncan

Typeset in Times 10/12pt by Leaper & Gard Ltd, Bristol
Printed in Great Britain by St Edmundsbury Press Ltd,
Bury St. Edmunds, Suffolk

ISBN 0 412 33940 4

British Library Cataloguing in Publication Data

Working with bilingual language disability.
  1. Bilingual children. Language disorders
  I. Duncan, Deirdre   II. Series
  618.92′855

  ISBN 0-412-33940-4

Library of Congress Cataloging in Publication Data

Working with bilingual language disability / edited by Deirdre M.
  Duncan.
      p.   cm. — (Therapy in practice)
  Bibliography: p.
  Includes index.
  ISBN 0-412-33940-4 (pbk.)
    1. Language disorders in children.   2. Bilingualism in children.
  I. Duncan, Deirdre M., 1952- .   II. Series
  RJ496.L35W67 1989
  618.92′855—dc19   88-30012
                                                          CIP

To all bilingual families
with language handicapped children

Contents

Contributors

Farat Ara was formerly a bilingual speech therapist, Central Manchester Health Authority.

Sarah Barnett was formerly a specialist speech therapist for bilingualism, City and Hackney Health Authority, London.

Deirdre Duncan is a research speech therapist for bilingualism, West Birmingham Health Authority.

Dorothy Gibbs was formerly a teacher and special needs liaison teacher, Ethnic Minority Support Service, Sandwell Local Education Authority, and is lecturer in multicultural studies, Henley College, Coventry.

Nita Madhani is a bilingual speech therapist specializing in special needs, Newham Health Authority, London.

Angela Roberts is a speech therapist and specializes in special needs, West Birmingham Health Authority.

Jane Stokes is a speech therapist for special units in the community, Tower Hamlets Health Authority, London.

Calla Thompson was formerly lecturer at the School of Speech Therapy, Manchester Polytechnic.

Preface

The decision to write this book was taken by a group of practising speech therapists who worked with bilingually language handicapped children in the UK. They formed a professional interest group called the Specific Interest Group in Bilingualism because of the need felt by speech therapists to have some forum for discussing the challenges posed by the assessment and treatment of the bilingually language handicapped.

In these regular discussion groups it became clear that similar experiences were encountered by all speech therapists working with these client populations up and down the country. They centred on managing the linguistic diversity, the need for developmental language information, the need for appropriate assessment protocols, the recruitment of bilingual staff and appreciating the positive perspective of working in this field.

In the UK the range of languages is extensive. Italian, Spanish, Portuguese, Greek, Turkish, Polish, Ukranian, Hong Kong Chinese, Vietnamese Chinese, Creole, Black English, Bengali, Gujerati and Panjabi cover the main ethnolinguistic groups. In the 1987 ILEA language census over 140 languages were recorded as being spoken in London.

In the face of this linguistic diversity, it was frustrating to decide where limited research resources should be invested for investigating the child language development of minority languages. The decision to start with the Panjabi and Bengali languages (Chapters 4 and 5) reflects more the language priority of the health districts involved in funding these projects rather than any nation-wide strategy. In fact the Linguistic Minorities Project (LMP) has shown that both are among the most spoken minority languages. The LMP was a government-sponsored research project which gathered detailed information about which languages other than English are in widespread use among children and adults in the UK.

The need for assessment procedures has long been recognized as a priority, while being riven with controversy. Tools and procedures are clearly needed to differentiate the quality of the language-learning problem and its severity in the bilingual or potentially bilingual child. The experiences, writings and practices of colleagues in bilingual societies in other countries have helped the development of assessments on formal and informal levels of bilingual performance (Chapter 8). Interestingly, the development has been away from translating English language assessments because it is linguistically and culturally unsatisfactory. Latterly, the move is towards developing bilingual assessments standardized on bilingual populations, and criteria-referenced procedures derived from language development information (Chapters 4–6).

It has become clear to the monoglot speech therapist working with bilingual clients that the recruitment of bilingual staff who share the home language of the client is fundamental and imperative. This is acknowledged in several countries, including the USA, Canada and the UK. However, there is a huge reluctance to provide the appropriate resources, whether it be creating specialist posts for work with bilingual clients or encouraging bilingual speakers to enter the professions – speech therapy, psychology and teaching – or to train as co-workers (Chapter 7). Without appropriate resources to access both languages of the bilingual client, speech therapists may not fulfil their professional responsibilities. Chapters 9 and 11 describe models of bilingual intervention, and Chapter 10 contains many examples of the need for a bilingual and bicultural approach when meeting the special educational needs of the child from a bilingual community.

The conventional format adopted in this book, setting out some theoretical models and empirical work in Part One, following in Part Two with practical applications and therapy models, emphasizes the view of the contributors. In the field of working with bilingualism, where many myths still abound, it is essential that clinical and educational remediation of the bilingual handicapped child be well-informed.

Some terminology used throughout the book may be controversial. For the purposes of clarification, the following points are noted: (a) the term 'the UK' is used to refer to the British Isles and is the region of reference for the working experience of this book; (b) the term 'practitioner' has been chosen to embrace many of the groups involved in working with bilingually language handicapped children such as speech therapists, psychologists, teachers, nursery nurses, teaching assistants, teachers of English as a second language (ESL), multicultural support workers and those involved in special education; (c) the pronoun 'she' is used throughout, which has a literary precedent in the field of bilingualism

(Skutnabb-Kangas, 1984); and (d) in the case studies fictitious names are used.

While we acknowledge that literary convention uses masculine pronouns, and that the statistical majority of language handicapped are male, we have chosen to use feminine pronouns throughout because the majority of practitioners working in this field are female.

Reference is made at various points through the book to the King's Fund. This is King Edward's Hospital Fund for London. It is an independent charity founded in 1897 and incorporated by act of Parliament. It seeks to encourage good practice and innovation in health care through research, experiment, education and direct grants.

Finally, reference is made in Chapters 9 and 11 to what some might see as parochial concerns, namely transport. These are included because they eloquently make the point that therapeutic success with the bilingually language impaired may not only depend on professional expertise, but also on accommodating cultural differences.

Through discussion and shared experiences the speech therapists in this forum appreciate and promote the positive perspective of working with the bilingually language handicapped. The bilingual client populations are viewed by some as a 'problem' because of their bilingualism, which stems largely from unawareness of the nature of bilingualism. It is more accurate to see the bilingual client populations as a challenge to the traditional monoglot perspective. This is not euphemistic jargon, but a fundamental concept which underpins the work in this book.

The parameters of the book are clearly defined. Our brief has been to reflect the experiences and the realities of working with bilingually language disabled children within a sound theoretical framework. These experiences and realities derive chiefly from clinical practice with the European and Asian ethnolinguistic populations in the UK. They embrace the issues facing all practitioners involved with this client population, such as teachers and psychologists, as well as students of these disciplines. The issues are assessment, language choice in therapy, developmental language information, therapy initiatives and bilingual staffing.

In a book of this size there are inevitable gaps, for example, language disability in the bilingually hearing impaired, dysfluency, phonology and therapy with the age-group of 3–6-year-olds. In fact this is a consequence not so much of lack of space, but of the lack of satisfactory clinical experiences which is, in turn, due to the lack of resources. It would be a happy continuation if this clinical vacuum were filled, and further chapters could be written in the near future. Furthermore, certain languages, such as Spanish and Welsh, which are important in the bilingualism debate, are not included here in any detail, and this is partly because both have been amply written about elsewhere (e.g. Miller, 1984; Abudarham, 1987). In addition, Spanish constitutes only a small part indeed of clinical experience in the UK. Welsh and Gaelic, although indigenous to the UK, occupy a different sociolinguistic status from the other minority languages in the country.

To conclude, although this book has been written by a group of authors, it is not an anthology. Considerable effort has been made to achieve cohesion while maintaining the essential variety of clinical experience in this field. By writing in some detail about this work it is hoped that other speech therapists and students will be encouraged to look for alternatives when organizing their own service and caseload. It is hoped that workers in associated fields will appreciate more fully the challenge of working with bilingualism. Most important, it is hoped that the specific experiences in this book may add to the more general body of knowledge of working with bilingual language disability in other countries, and to the wider field of development, disability and therapy in child language.

Deirdre M. Duncan

PART ONE

Theory and Research

1

Theory and Practice

Deirdre M. Duncan

INTRODUCTION

The importance of identifying and working with language impaired children from bilingual communities has long been recognized by those involved with this work. However, work with the bilingually language impaired is often regarded as a marginal aspect to the more general work with language disability. This is ironic since, on the theoretical side, bilingualism and second language acquisition (SLA) study has a respectable tradition in linguistic research.

It is the relationship between theory, empiricism/research and practice which is discussed in this chapter. This is achieved by looking at the research models available, and reviewing the methodological variations occurring in research which bear on interpreting findings. A brief comment on terminology is also given. Throughout the chapter the need for an informed theoretical and empirical concept of bilingualism is emphasized in order to understand the challenge of bilingualism.

THE CHALLENGE OF BILINGUALISM

Bilingualism as such does not constitute a problem. The majority of the world's population speaks more than one language. A society which is largely monolingual and monocultural, such as the British society 50 years ago, will demonstrate considerable inertia when absorbing influxes of peoples with different languages and cultures. This inertia may be compounded by the need to allocate resources to overcoming linguistic and cultural barriers. One of the challenges must be to overcome the social inertia and to find resources.

Those who say that bilingualism is a problem are usually monolingual, and argue from a lack of awareness of what bilingualism is. Any definition of bilingualism must include linguistic and cultural dimensions. The bilingual is not a 'monolingual speaker times two'; the bilingual has an integrated whole linguistic system which manifests in two languages. Bilingual speakers use these two languages in the two cultures within which they move, so causing language and culture to be inextricably bound. The implications of this concept are wide-ranging. Linguistically, the bilingual will offer a unique language profile which will have a bearing on developmental bilingual information, bilingual assessments and remediation. Socioculturally, there are implications for choice of language in therapy, and the emotional attitude and motivation of the client and family which, of course, will directly influence the success of therapy.

Each bilingual population is linguistically and culturally distinct. This is not to say that it is clinically distinct. The bilingual client population does not present with unique speech and language pathologies — although this could be debated in certain cases of language and phonology disorders. Their speech and language problems do not demand different principles of assessment and therapy from the monolingual population. The bilingually language handicapped population is distinct because it challenges the *application* of our principles and methods such as case-history taking, bilingual assessment, therapy through the mother tongue and counselling. We must look for ways which will enable us to apply our skills to meet the communication problems of this client group.

In the face of the challenge presented by the bilingually language impaired child, there seem to be three identifiable reactions: complacency, confusion and frustration. The complacent attitude towards the bilingually language handicapped must be seriously countered. It is expressed by sentiments such as: 'There are none in my district' or 'There are none on my caseload' or 'Most of them speak a bit of English'. No numbers, or low numbers, have never been accepted by any profession as sufficient reason for maintaining an ignorance about the therapy resources needed for satisfactorily managing a client group. The educational provision is there. There are lectures on bilingualism included in some training courses. Maybe this could be developed and supplemented by in-service training on racial awareness, as well as bilingualism and speech therapy?

Assimilation seemed to be an elegant solution to the 'problem' of non-English speaking people in the UK. However, it has since been shown to be morally dubious and sociologically unobtainable. The ethnolinguistic groups in the UK have shown that they are choosing to maintain their linguistic and cultural heritage through first and second generations by bringing up their children bilingually. So regardless of the amount of English spoken by the bilingual clients, it is crucial to access *both* of their languages.

Confusion is most probably felt by the majority of speech therapists towards achieving effective management of this client group. It is most commonly expressed in sentiments of being overwhelmed by the challenge and seeing no clear way forward to meet it, so that small client numbers justify monolingual intervention and large numbers are 'coped' with. Finding out alternative ways forward from multiracial and multidisciplinary discussion groups would be one solution.

The ultimate answer for those who see avenues for developing a satisfactory service for the bilingually language handicapped must be organizational. The feelings of frustration usually precipitated by challenging the limited resources of an overstretched budget can be resolved partly by departmental (re-)organization, and inter-departmental co-operation and support. Most of all, it depends on a fundamental change in sociopolitical attitudes which would release the necessary fiscal resources. Having discussed the need for the practitioner to meet the challenge of the bilingual client group positively, it is now necessary to consider the theory and research in bilingualism and SLA in order to appreciate how the theory informs clinical application.

'PURE' RESEARCH AND 'ACTION' RESEARCH

The practitioner should appreciate the complementary roles which the researcher and the clinician enjoy. There is a long-standing body of opinion which would like to see more practitioners participating in research. The polemic centres on the terms 'pure' research and 'action' research, that is Research and research!

Pure research refers to the traditional role of research which

5

seeks to challenge the plausibility of theories by investigating variables presented in different contexts, implementing rigorous scientific methodology. The classic practice of investigating is to isolate variables. This often makes research findings seem artificial, remote and difficult to apply. The onus is on practitioners to acquaint themselves with the relevant theory being investigated and to apply the findings appropriately. Often by appreciating the theoretical hypothesis underlying the research, the practitioner can attempt to explain and connect behaviours of the client which occur in a variety of contexts, particularly when working with the bilingual client.

Further, there is a great deal of research in the field of language development which can be applied to clinical and pedagogic language work. There are also studies which have particularly addressed themselves to certain problems and issues encountered in clinical practice.

Action research is more related to practical issues. It is defined as 'small-scale intervention in the functioning of the real world and close examination of its effects' (Halsey, 1972), and as 'on-the-spot procedure designed to deal with a concrete problem located in an immediate situation' (Cohen and Manion, 1986). In reviewing the role of action research, French (1987) states: 'The main aim of action research is ... to change practice or solve a particular problem within a specific practical context. The results may, however, not only help to solve practical problems, but also give insights that help to develop existing theory.' She goes on to note the disadvantages involved: 'action research lacks scientific rigour; the results cannot be easily generalised; there is little control over its subjects; and samples tend to be small and non-representative, criticism that could be levelled against most "naturalistic" research'. She concludes that it can contribute importantly to practice and theory.

It is crucial to remember that research and **therapy** are not interchangeable. They have distinct roles directed towards different ends. Therapy can never be a substitute for research because of the ethical considerations involved. Good research might make for very unethical therapy, for example, denying therapy to control groups of language handicapped children. However, therapy has been positively influenced by some of the scientific methods of research work. It should be standard practice for clinicians to assess objectively their work with clients, to hypothesize about the pathology and remediation strategies, and methodically to carry through these ideas and to record accurately the outcome. This is therapy and not research.

Thus there can be no doubt that the practitioner needs a sound theoretical framework in order to work most effectively with clients. Professional organization should allow her to work in 'pure' and 'action' research whenever possible. Some of the work in this book shows how this has been achieved in the field of speech therapy with language handicapped bilingual children.

Theories

One of the advantages of being a practitioner is that when it comes to theories and allegiances to schools of thought, one can be eclectic. That is not to argue that one works with one's head in the sand. It means that the practitioner has the facility to choose the theoretical framework which best interprets the current research findings and which is most appropriate to resolving the needs of the client(s).

People of many disciplines are working in the field of bilingualism, each developing a theory of second language acquisition within the parameters of their own discipline. These include applied linguistics, social psychology, sociolinguistics, psychology, neurolinguistics and education. They tend to function autonomously, publish in their respective journals and too infrequently share their work and ideas to move towards a more comprehensive view of the field.

It could be argued that the practitioner does not seek a theory about bilingualism and second language acquisition. Rather she wishes for more description about how bilinguals perform and how their languages develop, to build up a broad and varied picture of what can be expected from the bilingual person.

Although there is value in this point of view, data can remain idiosyncratic and infinitely variable unless global patterns are sought. As Lightbown (1984) has pointed out, there are huge collections of data and there seems little point in collecting more of the same. It is most important that patterns can be identified, against which hypotheses can be tested and tentative generalizations made, then paradigms and theories constructed and reconstructed in the light of new data and hypotheses. The process is cyclical. Since it is impossible to collect data for every conceivable language behaviour, theories enable predictions to be made about future possible behaviours.

The practitioner may also argue against the applicability of many research findings and theories because of the experimental nature and/or contrived situations from which the data derive. The relevance and application of research findings will continue to be hotly debated, and care must always be taken in generalizing research findings. What is fundamentally important is to maintain the integrity of the data, and to avoid mis-interpretation or over-interpretation, thus making the data subservient to a theory or a point of view.

The second language acquisition (SLA) literature is prolific. Before discussing the major findings and their application to work with bilingual children, it is necessary first to appreciate the methodological and disciplinary constraints which pepper the controversies and make generalizations problematic.

Methodology

The reason for looking at the methodological constraints and dilemmas in the research on bilingualism is to show that most of them are similar to the constraints acting in the classroom and clinic. Despite the fact that the studies are done by myriad disciplines, usually only dimly related to the discipline of the practitioner, she must take on board all the factors involved in working with the bilingual child.

Problems of data collection for assessment, analysis frameworks, aspects of language to investigate, and the differences and often uniqueness of the bilingual clients, all apply to classroom and clinic. There is a further constraint on the practitioner. The researcher usually has limited subjects and a generous supply of time. The opposite usually pertains to the practitioner.

This review also serves to show the range of problems confronting work with bilingualism; and the hazards of reaching simplistic conclusions.

Lightbown (1984) has compared the main differences in the methodology and aims of the disciplines involved in SLA research, and argued that research in the field of SLA should lead to the development of a scientific theory of language acquisition but was hampered by the diversity of disciplines involved. Against these two points, Ellis (1984) has argued that such a theory might not always be appropriate in SLA studies, and rather than regard the diversity of methodology as limiting, one can view these various approaches as throwing a different light on second language acquisition. This should be seen as a considerable advantage; no single discipline would have the range or the funding to do so much research.

Language

Most of the SLA research has been carried out on the acquisition of English. There are some studies which look at other languages (e.g. Johnston and Slobin, 1979; Zobl, 1982). It is a recognized need in the field that other additional languages be studied if generalizations about second language acquisition are to have credibility.

Aspects of language

Most of the SLA studies have selected one aspect of language to investigate. It has usually been syntax, reflecting the general preoccupation in psycholinguistic research in the last decade. Originally many studies investigated only morphology, but recently phrasal and clausal structures have also been investigated. There are some studies which have chosen to look at vocabulary development in the bilingual child (Rescorla and Okuda, 1984; Meara, 1984), and others have looked at phonology (Munro, 1985). Semantics is under-represented in bilingual research studies; and recent investigations (see Chapter 6) are attempting to correct this omission. Pragmatics and language function have received some attention (Chesterfield and Chesterfield, 1985) and are on the agenda for more research.

Linked with pragmatic aspects of language are the sociolinguistic investigations of bilingualism. They look at **diglossia** and **code-switching** in bilingual language use (Chana and Romaine, 1984): diglossia is the functional distribution of two or more languages or language varieties within a speech community, and code-switching is moving from one language to another within the same conversation.

Data collection

There are numerous ways of collecting language data, with ranging degrees of compatibility and inherent difficulty. There seems to be little controversy over the compatibility of data collected from longitudinal and cross-sectional methods (Chomsky, 1969; Andersen, 1977); although there are fewer longitudinal studies (Leopold, 1970; Wode, 1978).

There is more controversy surrounding testing vs. naturalistic data collection. The discrete point testing used in many studies, particularly in morphological studies (Krashen, Long and Scarcella, 1979, SLOPE), is strongly criticized because it removes the linguistic features from their functional context and places them in isolation. The artificiality of such language use, limiting the language contexts, must therefore limit performance. Krashen (1978) argues against the fact that test results may be artefacts of the test, and claims that spontaneous speech data reflect the same morphological order.

Data collected naturalistically avoids the inherent problems of artificiality posed by testing. However, it takes longer to collect the data, and there may be difficulties of replication. Testing is relatively quick and replicable, but the price is highly selective and possibly artificial data. Because of these differences, the two methods are often adopted to meet different research needs. Testing is usually used on large numbers of subjects, while naturalistic data collection is used with small numbers.

Many studies have investigated the development of a second language on expressive language performance, while others (e.g. White, 1985) have based their conclusions about second language acquisition on work done on the analysis of comprehension and grammatical judgement tasks. The extent to which the results from these two types of experiment are compatible must remain controversial albeit very interesting.

Finally, most controversy centres on the compatibility — or lack of compatibility — of results obtained through literacy tasks and oracy tasks. It must be argued that speaking and writing, although deriving from a common language source, actually recruit different skills in their execution. Further, there is the variable of education/ schooling to be taken into account. There are studies which have obtained their data through literacy tasks and then interpreted their conclusions within the framework of hypotheses developed from second language oracy data. However, it is a very contentious area and recurs in the discussion about semilingualism.

ANALYSIS

The method of analysing the data reflects the concept of language development and bilingualism, and is often determined by the method of data collection. Many studies of monolingual language acquisition and SLA base their analysis on a comparison of the subjects' emerging language with adult target language (TL). There are drawbacks in such a comparison with developing monolinguals and more serious issues involved when comparing SLA with monolingual adult language. The fundamental problem in the comparison is avoiding comparing the 'real' with the 'ideal'. Alderson (1980) has argued that often bilingual subjects were compared with idealized expectations of the target language behaviour, which might not have been achievable, even by monolingual adult speakers. He argues, as do others (e.g. Martin-Jones and Romaine, 1986), for the development of language baselines drawn from the relevant populations against which language performance can be compared — e.g. drawing up the TL of monolingual children at differing ages, and most important, the TL of bilingual children and adults. The concept underlying comparing second language learners with the TL of monolingual adults is that the aim of second language acquisition should be to acquire the second language to the same degree of proficiency and quality as the monolingual. Clearly, this is a controversial idea and such a premiss would be hotly disputed by many; it is discussed later.

Some analyses are conducted on an item-by-item procedure, where they are marked right/wrong, present/absent. This reflects language development as being correct or erroneous and leaves no room to show the developmental dimension of SLA. Such procedures are usually determined by the nature of the data collection, for example, testing — particularly **cloze testing**, which is the removal of a word at regular, predicted intervals for the subject to supply. Other analyses, usually of naturalistic data, attempt to

11

capture the *sui generis* nature of the emerging language, analysing it descriptively rather than prescriptively. The studies with simultaneous bilinguals often use this analysis. Finally, depending on the aspect of language being investigated, phonology, syntax, semantics, vocabulary, function and the detail of the analysis will vary respectively.

SUBJECTS

A great deal of experimental research is conducted on sequential bilinguals — that is, subjects who have acquired to some degree their first language before starting to acquire their second language. These subjects vary in **age**: research (Krashen *et al.*, 1979, Fathman, 1975) has shown that age is an important variable in the acquisition of second language, in as much as children and adults will acquire the same basic English morphology in about the same time span, although adults are marginally quicker. Adults will be slower to progress to more complex structures. It is also recognized that there are influences operating in adult learners, such as motivational and cognitive factors, which do not seem to be so influential in child learners; Krashen's Monitor Theory (1981) is a good example of this. When making comparisons between studies, it must be borne in mind that some studies will be done with undergraduate and graduate students (White, 1985; Mazurkewich, 1983), while others are conducted with pre-school and primary school aged children (Dulay and Burt, 1974; Nwokah, 1984).

Finally, in the broader field of bilingualism, there are studies which look at the development of two languages in simultaneous bilingualism. Simultaneous bilinguals are those who from the onset of language acquisition are exposed to two languages and are required to communicate in both. It could be argued that these studies (Volterra and Taeschner, 1978; Redlinger and Park, 1980) are not happily compatible with the studies of sequential bilinguals. Simultaneous bilinguals are not subject to the same variables as are the sequential bilinguals. That is not to say that the process might not be the same. The challenge must be to find out what are the core similarities in the process of bilingual language development across all the factors.

IMPLICATIONS

One of the fundamental linguistic findings is that early emerging morphology and syntax of English seem to develop in a similar pattern in both first and second language English, in primary school aged children, with mother tongue and gender not presenting as significant variables. This suggests that descriptive development profiles of the structure of first language English could be used to chart the morpho-syntactic development of L2 English. Naturalistic data would be required and profiles, such as LARSP (Crystal, Garman and Fletcher, 1976), could be used.

Three points are needed to qualify this procedure. First, LARSP is a profile of syntax structure only. Secondly, as with monolingual children, account would need to be taken of the bilingual child's other language systems (vocabulary, semantics, functions and phonology) in English. Thirdly, there will be always be idiosyncrasies in the individual's development of the sequence of features whether the child is monolingual or bilingual (Wode, 1978). The profile will reflect the distribution of the morpho-syntactic features used by the children in their developing English language system.

This finding also implies that the aspects of therapy in L2 English for the bilingual language impaired child which involve grammatical structure could be based on the developmental framework of first language English structures. Findings from the other aspects of language development are necessary to put this suggestion in a total bilingual perspective.

There is little research information about the assessment of comprehension of additional language. Grammatical judgement tasks are not appropriate for the purposes of most practitioners who seek to determine how much the child is understanding of the linguistic environment rather than to gain insights about the influence of one language upon another.

One cannot assess one language through the medium of another — i.e. translating language tests. The arguments against doing so are very strong. Most language tests have a rationale deriving from the linguistic systems of that language. Translations will not assess the structures which are pertinent to, and the hallmark of, the other language. The issues surrounding bilingual language assessment are taken up more fully in Chapter 8.

The influence of the mother tongue on the second language

is being continually refined. It is most certainly not a simple 1:1 interference relationship of one structure upon another, as was once thought. It may be idiosyncratic to the child or it may depend on formal/developmental structural congruencies (Zobl, 1980) or it may be contingent upon context, semantic and pragmatic factors. At best, the relationship is ambiguous (see Chapter 2).

With regard to teaching the additional language to developing bilinguals, findings have shown (Ellis, 1981) that structured formal input which is not in line with the subject's developmental acquisition level may have an adverse and detrimental effect on the development of the second language. Furthermore, it may have adverse effects on the development of the mother tongue. The implications for the clinician and educationist are that intervention and formal instruction should be preceded by careful assessment in all areas of both languages, so that language stimulation programmes for potentially normal developing language, and language intervention programmes for remediating deviant or delayed bilingual language patterns, should select developmentally appropriate structures for the child/children receiving the programmes (see Chapters 9 and 11).

Following from this is the finding that developing bilingual children seem to acquire more language through peer interaction and groupwork than through 'teacher fronted' work (Long and Porter, 1985). Furthermore, teachers seem more likely to refer bilingual children for speech therapy on the grounds of pragmatic dysfunctions, rather than for grammatical problems, and those children seem to have more serious remediation problems (Damico, Oller and Storey, 1983). These findings about the functional aspects of language suggest that language work should take place in the most functional and meaningful contexts for the bilingual child, if possible including group dynamics.

Associated with these points are the affective variables (see Chapter 2) involved in language acquisition. It has been shown that just as with monolingual language acquisition, the motivation and emotional set of the child towards acquiring the second language will be very important. Two implications follow from this. First, the language learning environment, whether it be classroom or clinic, should be motivation enhancing towards the second language. Secondly, it is possible to conclude that a non-talking minority first language (L1) child in the L2 class may be language impaired. Assessment in both L1 and L2 would reveal her language performance bilingually. A depressed profile in only L2 would indicate acquisition problems in only that language, not a bilingual problem and not a language learning problem *per se*. So it seems that providing a happy, non-pressurized language environment is the optimum for developing language in the bilingual child. This includes allowing the child to choose which language she prefers to communicate in — e.g. L1 to her L1 peers and L2 to her L2 peers and teachers.

It hardly needs research findings to show that the development of the second language will depend on the exposure that the child has to that language. Yet this is not quite so axiomatic as it may appear; there are many other sociolinguistic variables which influence the development of both languages of the developing bilingual child. In the UK social class is an important variable in the development of English in the monolingual (Wheldall and Martin, 1977). This factor is less obtrusive in the development of L2 English among Panjabi speaking children in the UK (Wheldall *et al.*, 1987). This is partly because of the problems encountered in trying to match social class register with social groupings in the ethnolinguistic population. Pehaps this is so in other countries?

A matrix of influential sociolinguistic factors has been identified (Duncan *et al.*, 1985), which includes the area of origin in the respective countries, length of residence and establishment in the present country, and language status and attitudes to the L1 and L2 in the home, community and school. The interplay of these factors seems to have influenced the bilingual language development of the Panjabi children in the study, in that a substantial minority of them performed better in L2 English than in their L1 Panjabi, on an assessment of expressive grammatical structure. All of the children showed that both languages continued to develop over time. These factors reinforce the notion that bilingual language development develops to meet the needs of the communicative environment of the child. It underlines the fact that assessment, therapy and management must meet the bilingual needs of the child involved.

This, then, concludes the brief overview of some of the theoretical and empirical work and its applications to working with bilingually language handicapped children. The final part of the chapter deals with the issue of terminology in the field and its appropriateness.

TERMINOLOGY

Throughout the literature the area of study is referred to, for the most part, as **second language acquisition** (SLA). There is a controversy about the accuracy and appropriateness of the term 'second language' in the clinical and educational spheres because it seems to imply non-native, and thereby inferior, language competence, and language inadequacy. With simultaneous bilinguals, using the term 'second language' acquisition is obviously inaccurate and inappropriate since both the speaker's languages are acquired simultaneously.

Sequential bilinguals acquire their first language in the home from infancy and then start in a major way the development of their other (second) language, and the language of the majority community, on entry into formal education, at around 3–5 years of age. It is arguable that it can still be regarded as their *second* language ten, twenty or more years later, when they will most probably perform functionally similarly to a native speaker.

In the older sequential bilingual who started to acquire the second language as a teenager or adult, the term 'second language' might possibly apply. It would be necessary to investigate more fully the linguistic abilities of such a speaker, bearing in mind primarily the functional use of that language and the 'success' achieved in that domain. This is a knotty problem and cannot be resolved on the basis of accent or vocabulary counts.

Thus, if only one group of bilinguals could possibly be regarded as 'second language' speakers, then we might be best advised to look for more accurate and appropriate terminology for this linguistic behaviour such as mother-tongue/additional language speakers.

The nature of bilingualism is discussed further in Chapter 2. However, this brief discussion of terminology shows how misconceptions may develop when 'shorthand' terms are used. Despite the pitfalls involved, the terms L1 and L2 will be used throughout the book, in line with most of the literature, because they are recognized as the 'industry standard'.

CONCLUSION

This introductory chapter has sought to give a bird's eye view of the topic of bilingualism as it pertains to practitioners, whether they are speech therapists, teachers, psychologists or students. The importance of a theoretical framework has been noted and the methodological differences in research discussed; some practical implications and applications have been derived and the challenges which working with bilingual language disability present have been highlighted. An attempt has been made to show that for the conscientious and eclectic practitioner there should be no chasms between theory, empiricism and practice.

The following chapters in the book take up and elucidate many of the points and issues raised in this chapter. Furthermore, it is hoped that they maintain the idea that good and successful intervention with the bilingually language impaired can best be achieved by a sound understanding of the linguistic and cultural nature of bilingualism.

2

Issues in Bilingualism Research

Deirdre M. Duncan

INTRODUCTION

The issues addressed in the research into bilingualism are often common to those of first language development. In other ways they are discrete. It is important to appreciate which issues are shared and which are unique in order to define more sharply the nature of bilingualism, which is imperative for the practitioner working with language impairment. Much of the ignorance and inaccuracies which underlie the layman's concept of bilingualism will prevent the practitioner from offering appropriate assessment and management. Furthermore, failing to appreciate the similarities and differences between monolingual and bilingual language development can only lead to frustration for all concerned.

This chapter aims to offer a working definition of bilingualism, to discuss the sociocultural issues involved and their practical implications, and to discuss the linguistic theories of second language acquisition and their relevance to clinical and pedagogic work. Finally, the controversial notion of semilingualism will be touched on.

DEFINING BILINGUALISM

As the literature on bilingualism grows so does the number and variety of definitions of bilingualism and the bilingual. These have been documented elsewhere (Abudarham, 1987). In discussions of nomenclature it is possible to miss seeing the wood for the trees. So briefly, the issue which will be discussed here is that concerning the situations creating bilingualism which generate these definitions.

Foreign language

Some would argue that any knowledge of another language would constitute a degree of bilingualism, including, for example, that at the holiday phrase-book level. This seems a very contentious claim and would occupy a fairly extreme position on the scale of definitions of bilingualism.

Moving along the scale are definitions concerning those who have learned a foreign language, that is a language not generally spoken in their mother-country and learnt as a school subject. Many who have experienced this would be reluctant to call themselves bilingual, even while they were learning the foreign language, and would be even more reluctant several years later when they may have forgotten most of it. Those who go on to study the foreign language at tertiary level, using it in their work, would be very proficient in the language. They probably could be called bilingual, although they might prefer to describe themselves as being 'speakers of another language' rather than being 'bilingual'. In other words, it could be said that from one perspective there seems to be more than levels of proficiency involved in being bilingual.

Second language

There are those who start their learning of a language as a school subject. Then they emigrate to a country where that language is used as the first language, and continue to develop it in a very different way.

This non-native speaking population usually creates two linguistic environments for itself. One is among their own community where they speak their mother tongue among adults and to their children. The second linguistic environment will be in their second language (L2) with the majority community. Some immigrant adults, such as older women, will rarely enter this L2 community and will learn very little of the host country's language. Many of the adults will learn the majority culture language in order to meet the communicative demands made by work, commerce or their children's schools. The children will begin to acquire the L2 as they enter more into the majority community, usually on entrance to formal school education.

This is the situation for many ethnolinguistic communities, for example in the UK, the USA, Canada, Australia and West Germany. Many of these people may not be very proficient in certain senses in the language of the host country, yet they constitute a population which is called 'bilingual'.

There are other examples where a (foreign) language school subject may become a second language. In certain areas, such as French Canada or Wales, as minority communities win the right to conduct education in their own first language (L1), children will be formally exposed to two languages. For these speakers one of the languages will function, and have communicative demands made on it, mainly or only within the school.

There are many situations which give rise to people learning two languages, but not necessarily all will become bilingual. It seems to be more than simply the knowledge, or some knowledge, of two or more languages. There needs to be a dimension of communicative demand. The person needs to be in a situation where both languages are continually needed for effective living.

To summarize, the most suitable working definition would be one which tries to embrace the linguistic, communicative and sociocultural aspects of the task facing the person developing in a bilingual environment. It is important that the clinician bears these three aspects in mind when working with the child from a minority language background whose language learning processes are impaired. Linguistically she must aim to assess and intervene in both languages of the child; she must try to offer language intervention which meets the communicative demands made on the child and which the child wishes to make on herself in both language environments; and she must appreciate with the family the sociocultural importance of both languages for the successful future communication of the emerging bilingually handicapped child.

This seems adequately to describe the bilingual populations under discussion in this book, and to be the definition most useful to clinicians and educationists.

Finally, it has to be said that each bilingual person is unique in her bilingualism, and that bilingual populations are different one from another. So, although for the purposes of brevity bilingualism and bilingual populations will be referred to, the heterogeneity of the phenomenon must be remembered. This will now be discussed in greater detail.

SOCIOCULTURAL ISSUES

Language change

The heterogeneity of bilingual populations will vary mainly because of intra-language variability. This variability is caused by large-scale influences from the majority language on the minority language. Thus, at phonological, morphological, syntactic and lexical levels, the minority language changes from the standard form to create a unique language variation.

This can happen to a greater or lesser extent. In its advanced form the unique variety is called a **contact dialect** (Haugen, 1977) and may be incomprehensible to standard speakers of the language. In the UK an example of this is Jamaican English, which differs sufficiently from Creole because of the large influence of English to constitute a unique language variety.

Less extreme examples are found in many minority languages and they are documented elsewhere (Brent-Palmer, 1979). Panjabi, as a minority language, differs in the various countries where it is spoken. For example, in Kenya it has been influenced by Swahili as well as English. In the UK, Panjabi will be influenced by the regional lexical and morphological differences. Most of the influences from English on Panjabi and Bengali in the UK seem to be in the domain of lexis and coinage of terms. This is in line with observations of other languages in their first stages of contact (Acosta-Belan, 1975, in Brent-Palmer, 1979). There may also be morphological and syntactic changes occurring. This requires more research.

Further, many minority language speakers may not speak a standard form of the language, but rather a rural, urban or 'old form' dialect. Examples include Sylhet Bengali, Mirpur Panjabi, Cypriot Greek, Cypriot Turkish and the *dialetti* of northern and southern Italy (Linguistic Minorities Project, 1985), as well as the historically older forms of French which may be spoken in Canada.

Cultural use of language

Discourse

Language is used differently in different cultures and subcultures. Different groups use different discourse styles. Labov's (1972) work has shown that the use of different language patterns and discourse styles reflects class differences and subculture distinctions rather than implying linguistic or cognitive deficits.

Research suggests that there may be two main discourse styles: the inductive approach and the deductive; a similar distinction can be drawn for cognitive styles, referred to as the **relational** and **analytical** respectively. Briefly, the **inductive** relational style involves making concrete statements from which fundamental assumptions are inferred, while the **deductive/analytical** style involves stating propositions and drawing inferences from them.

It seems that cultural groups will reflect one approach in their use of language. For example, West Indian and East Indo-Pakistani groups, as well as lower-class UK children, reflect the inductive/relational style, while middle-class Anglo-Americans, North Americans and upper-middle-class children in the UK reflect the deductive/analytical approach, as documented in Brent-Palmer (1979).

Literacy

Other forms of language use will be regarded differently in different cultures and subcultures. In the middle and upper classes of European and Euro-American societies literacy is given a primacy which is encouraged by parents of (their) children from a young age. By contrast, cultures which encourage face-to-face interaction maintain rich oracy traditions with literacy having a low profile. Again, these sociolinguistic distinctions cut along ethnic and social class lines.

Language functions

Language has many functions and social cultures place different emphases on them. Once again, these differences are reflected in ethnic and class groupings and are among the distinguishing features of those communities.

Language functions can be summarized as follows: to inform (referential), to learn and solve problems (heuristic), to express emotions (expressive), to persuade others to do something (manipulative), to demonstrate social identity and status (integrative), to discipline social behaviour (social control) and to develop language for its own sake (aesthetic) (Halliday 1973; and see also Chapter 6).

Research shows that functions such as the aesthetic and expressive functions are characteristics of societies which are less technologically advanced, and also lower-class urban subcultures such as black ghetto Americans, some south-east Asians and many lower-class European children. On the other hand, the heuristic, referential, social control and integrative functions appear more in the language of the upper classes of the more technical, literate societies. The clinical and pedagogic implications of these findings are considerable.

Macro-social effects on the individual: sociopolitical issues

It is impossible to discuss sociocultural aspects of bilingualism without referring to the wider sociopolitical backcloth against which the bilingual communities and bilingual individuals must function. In the above discussion there has been no attempt to place values on the sociolinguistic behaviour of different cultural groups. Yet one of the key features of sociolinguistic change is the ascribing of such values. In almost all bilingual societies the languages are differentiated along sociopolitical lines, where one language will be dominant — usually that belonging to the majority or the politically more powerful community — and the other language(s) of the minority or less powerful communities is subordinated. One possible result of this 'linguistic oppression' (Trudgill, 1974) may be the erasing of subordinate languages from the linguistic map of the society. Such an outcome is usually the result of the machinations, direct or subtle, of sociopolitical mechanisms. The dominant language group will have the systems — legislative and economic — to determine the resources which could maintain or undermine the existence of the subordinate language(s). Lack of official recognition of a language usually means that that language cannot be used by its speakers for social, educational or economic advancements.

This is the observed experience in countries with a long-standing tradition of bilingualism. The challenge for the recognition of bilingualism as a new social phenomenon is felt more keenly by countries, such as the UK and Australia, which are experiencing the establishment of large, new ethnolinguistic communities.

The linguistic minority groups, and the dominant language groups, are often acutely aware of the different status the languages occupy. This may entail stigmatizing the minority languages and cultures, and may be interpreted as another strategy for maintaining the superiority of the dominant language.

Assimilation has often been the path to linguistic and cultural identity loss; consequently, many ethnolinguistic communities will guard their linguistic and cultural heritage, creating distinct sub-societies, and seeking more linguistic rights, such as mother-tongue teaching and educational recognition of the minority language skills.

The micro-social effects on the individual

It is clear that with such macro-social factors, the emerging bilingual child may absorb some of the feelings of 'conflict' and 'stigma' about the languages she is being exposed to, and reflect them in her own language behaviour. The most common place for experiencing these tensions is usually the initial formal introduction to the dominant/second language. The child may experience 'cultural dislocation', that is a culture gap between the familiar culture of the home and the non-familiar culture behaviour experienced in school.

Research suggests that children learning L2 may adopt different strategies for handling the feelings of 'stigma' attached to their L1. One is maintaining a silence in their mother tongue (i.e. concealment), and the other is maintaining a silence in their mother tongue to the wider group of peers, yet revealing their L1 to a smaller group of fellow speakers (i.e. concealment and in- and out-group membership). Silence and passive acquiescence is a feature of behaviour of many school entrants with minority L1 languages.

Language of school

One of the key issues debated by educationists concerns the language(s) of the educational system. In the UK the debate has been opened up considerably with the passing of the EEC Directive in the late 1970s making it a legal requirement for mother-tongue teaching to be available to all ethnolinguistic minorities. The Linguistic Minorities Project (LMP) (1985) notes that many communities have had mother-tongue classes operating for some time, often associated with the communities' religious centre — e.g. Italian in the Catholic Church, Urdu in the Mosque.

There are cognitive-linguistic issues involved in the debate about bilingual education, which will be dealt with later. The socio-cultural issue is mainly that of mother-tongue teaching and maintenance. Some ethnolinguistic groups, particularly the larger ones, for example, the Urdu and Panjabi speaking communities in the UK wish to see more integration of the teaching of their language into the educational system. Among other things, they would like their language taught as formal curriculum subject. Given the earlier discussion about dialectal variation and language change, it is clear that there is much debate about what constitutes the mother-tongue language for some bilingual children. Teaching the standard form of the L1 might not be their mother tongue — e.g. the *dialetti* of Italy vs Standard Italian (LMP, 1985). Mother-tongue literacy is a further, separate issue.

There seems to be wider support for the argument for having mother-tongue teachers in the early years of schooling. This would attempt to cope with the cultural dislocation and 'concealment' phenomena, and would encourage conceptual development through the mother tongue at a crucial learning period in the development of the child.

IMPLICATIONS

The clinical and educational implications from the findings of these investigations are considerable. Three main areas present themselves. First, and most fundamental, is the issue of the effect of macro-social factors on the L2 individual's behaviour. In appreciating these factors the practitioners raises their own consciousness about cultural, linguistic and racist attitudes. Without this appreciation, successful rapport with the client group and with individual children and their families becomes very difficult.

The second important implication bears on mother-tongue assessment. Dialectal variation and contact dialect illustrate how misleading it can be to rely solely on standard forms of language description in assessing the child's mother tongue. Furthermore, bilingual co-workers should be aware of possible variations from the standard form when they are assessing. There are implications, too, for the methodology used in assessment techniques, bearing in mind the different cultural attitudes towards discourse, language functions and literacy which may well exist between clinician and client.

Finally, there are implications for remediation. The culture gap experienced on entry to school may be experienced by the child in clinic. Additional pressure may be placed on the child who has been used to enjoying learning experiences through peer inter-action, and who is now expected to develop and learn through child–adult interaction. Language clinicians may have to alter radically their traditional remediation models with the bilingual client group in the light of this information.

Theoretical linguistic framework for the acquisition of second language

One of the perennial concerns of language research is the develop-ment of a theory of language acquisition. This research and its relevance to bilingualism will be discussed, together with its bear-ing on clinical and pedagogic work.

It seems to be widely accepted that there is an innate facility for the acquisition of language based on a cerebral and physiological predisposition. There seems to be a 'blueprint' (Aitchison, 1976) in the brain for language acquisition — a language acquisition device — which constrains the emergence of language features. Some aspects of language seem to be more 'tightly wired' than others, that is the rule systems or processes or constraints for syntax and phonology seem to be more readily identified and described than for semantics and pragmatics.

The **Acquisition–Learning Hypothesis** for second language development is based on this premiss, in that it accepts that language, particularly first language, is largely acquired in a non-conscious way through neurolinguistic facilities. It further propounds that teaching/learning may have an effective role in second language development, whereas they do not seem to play a part in first language acquisition (Brown, 1973; Newport *et al.*, 1977). Chomskean ideas about core and peripheral grammar are the theoretical framework for this hypothesis.

Core grammar is the set of linguistic universals which are the basis of all languages. This is not to be confused with Greenberg's language universals, which are cross-linguistic similarities such as word order and categorial harmony. **Peripheral grammar** is the acquisition of language-specific rules which modify the language universals in the core grammar. To test this theory some research has looked at the syntactic rules of the first and second languages of certain bilinguals — i.e. contrastive linguistic analysis — to identify rules which differ, in order to investigate the establishment of these rules in the second language. It predicts that second language acquisition should move from the core grammar to developing a peripheral grammar by setting new parameters for specific rules. For example, it is hypothesized that core grammar does not contain subject pronouns, indeed there are many peripheral grammars which reflect this constraint — e.g. the pro-drop parameter (Panjabi and Spanish). English requires subject pronouns and so has to set a pronoun parameter in its peripheral grammar. When this rule is investigated in emerging second language English speakers with L1 Spanish, the pro-drop parameter is maintained, which seems to support this hypothesis for second language acquisition (White, 1985).

The implications of this hypothesis for clinical and pedagogic work is that with appropriate linguistic assessment of the second language learner's English and contrastive linguistic analysis of the learner's first language, input in terms of teaching and learning can be maximized.

This hypothesis, then, seems to be similar to one put forward in the late 1950s (Lado, 1957), called the **Contrastive Analysis Hypothesis** (CAH). This hypothesis argued that second language developed in the context of the first language, and that the contrastive linguistic analysis of the first and second languages' grammars could explain and *predict* the 'errors' of the second language development.

The main difference between the Acquisition–Learning Hypothesis and the CAH is that the former is placed within the broader framework of linguistic theory relating to language acquisition in general, whereas the CAH derives from a linguistic analysis procedure and has been linked with behaviourist notions of language learning.

It was to disprove the CAH that researchers in the 1970s

investigated the language development of young emerging bilingual children (Dulay and Burt, 1974; Fathman, 1975; Krashen, Long and Scarcella, 1979). By looking at the fairly restricted field of morphological development they showed that second language acquisition of English followed a broadly similar pattern to that of first language English. A great deal more research has since gone on to support this **Natural Order Hypothesis**, and to modify it by accepting that there seem to be individual idiosyncrasies (Wode, 1978), that there have only been a few languages investigated, and that although second language English does not develop in an identical way to first language English, it seems to develop in a predictable way regardless of the mother tongue of the learner.

The implications for intervention with this hypothesis is that teaching/learning of second language syntax is redundant, just as in normal first language acquisition. This may be satisfactory for young bilinguals, but it does not resolve the problem of non-target grammatical forms, such as fossilization, which may occur in the second language of the older emerging bilingual. Further, it fails to account for certain conscious forms of language development, which follow from self-monitoring and self-correction of both the spoken and written forms of the second language. This is usually a feature of meta-linguistic maturity and is observed in the adolescent and adult learner. This possible explanation of second language development is known as the **Monitor Hypothesis** (Krashen, 1981).

There remains the problem of explaining the non-target grammar forms — i.e. those structures which are not acceptable grammar forms in young emerging bilinguals. The Natural Order Hypothesis argues that these are a product of language development mechanisms, and that most second language non-target grammar forms are similar to developing first language forms; indeed, this is often, but not always, the case. On the other hand, the Acquisition–Learning Hypothesis has no problem accounting for non-target forms, but seems unable to account for their selective nature.

An hypothesis put forward by Zobl (1980) in the structuralist tradition postulates that there may be two linguistic axes — a formal and a developmental — to consider when attempting to explain the selective nature of non-target grammar forms, that is specifically contact-induced language change. Non-target grammar forms can be predicted by structural incongruities between the first and second languages, yet their emergence into the second language may be constrained by the developmental axis of the sequence of emergence of features in both the first and second language. So although there may be theoretically possible transfer structures, such as adjective agreement (e.g. 'reds shoes'), they never occur in normal second language English development because this morphological rule is later acquired in languages requiring adjective concord rather than the non-concord rule in English. Consequently, for contact-induced language forms to emerge in the second language there must be linguistic synchrony along formal and developmental axes of the first and second languages.

One of the clinical implications is that any productive use of non-target grammar forms by a young second language learner which challenges this **Selectivity Hypothesis** could be a differentially diagnostic feature between delay and deviance in second language acquisition. More information about the developmental sequences of different mother tongues is obviously needed.

A more popular hypothesis which focuses on the semantic and contextual factors involved in the second language is the **Input Hypothesis** (Krashen, 1981). 'The Input Hypothesis postulates that we acquire by understanding ... language that contains input containing structures that are a bit beyond the acquirer's level.' (Krashen, 1982.) That is, comprehensible input moves the learner's language system from i to $i + 1$. Krashen goes on to claim 'That the "best" input should not be "gramatically sequenced", that is that it should not deliberately aim at $i + 1$ .... Acquirers will receive comprehensible input if they are in situations involving genuine communication ...' (p. 59). Indeed, the importance of understanding through semantics, context and knowledge of the world has long been recognized in the development of first language — namely, in the semantic primacy principle (Beheydt, 1984).

However, despite a considerable degree of support among practitioners, the Input Hypothesis has been criticized on several grounds. Studies of simplified input, such as 'motherese' (e.g. Newport, Gleitman and Gleitman, 1977), suggest that it is unlikely that there is a syntax-teaching component in this talk form since there is no correlation between the frequency of the mothers' grammatical structures and the acquisition patterns of the children. It is also strongly criticized for its inherent confusions about theoretical linguistics.

Thus the exclusivity of Krashen's claim challenges ideas held in other hypotheses that language acquisition may be caused by the inherent dynamic of language acquisition; that is, rule acquisition may be provoked when a linguistic stimulus — trigger — challenges the learner's grammar because it is not understood and thus cannot be processed by the present grammar. For example, the sentence: 'The car was kissed by the giant' will seriously challenge the grammar of a learner who has not acquired the passive. Such a sentence would be interpreted as 'The car kissed the giant'. Knowledge of the world (cars are unable to kiss) could provoke the acquisition of the passive through the use of 'by' before the agent; hence 'The car kissed by the giant' would be a satisfactory rule acquisition. The acquisition of the auxiliary in such a context would seem to require different triggers since auxiliaries have little semantic content. Current research suggests that linguistic reorganization may provoke, as a linguistic trigger, further reorganization (White, 1987). Further, there is the evidence from normal first language development where the child will generate rules which will not have been part of the input (Brown, 1973; Randell, 1985).

The pedagogic implications of the Input Hypothesis are that second language acquisition is most effective in a linguistic environment which is optimally understood by the learner. This would argue against classes of children of differing language levels, which is unfortunately often the case in the early years of school. It would also argue against any formal language instruction for normal second language learners. Of course, for non-normal development 'more of the same' input would not be appropriate. The challenge presented would be that of the Acquisition–Learning Hypothesis, which would be to identify the language structures in the learner's system and to note the aspects of input which interact with them. The issue about which language(s) the assessment and intervention should take place in would then need to be tackled.

There are also affective variables which might influence the development of the second language. They are prevalent enough in second language learners to have formed the basis of an hypothesis, namely the **Affective Filter Hypothesis** (Dulay and Burt, 1977). Low anxiety, high motivation, and the self-confidence and self-esteem of the acquirer all positively influence second language acquisition (Krashen, 1981). If these affective variables are in a less than optimal state, then it seems that there may be a filter inhibiting the effective operation of language acquisition.

Implications for differential diagnosis follow from this hypothesis. An emerging bilingual child presenting with noticeable second language delay may not require linguistic intervention, but possibly some form of counselling or a change of environment (see Chapter 11).

Finally, there are cognitive factors which affect language acquisition, namely conceptual development and psycholinguistic factors, and they seem to influence first and second language development differently. The conceptual aspect has to do with Piagetian ideas about the development of concepts which may underpin certain language structures, for example, vocabulary acquisition, notions of probability reflected in modality and contingency in subordination. In normal first language acquisition conceptual development and language development progress in synchrony. In second language development they are usually not in synchrony because the conceptual development of the learner will be at a more advanced stage than that of the emerging second language structures. This presents certain frustrations in input, for example, for the teacher in the classroom, and in using didactic materials — as well as in output, for example, the level of syntactic and semantic structures of the second language learner may not facilitate the expression of certain ideas.

Psycholinguistic factors refer to those cerebral and physical facilities which enable language use. They include auditory memory, attention, sequencing and motor development. In the first language they appear to restrain the Chomskean hypothesis of language acquisition because they are subject to maturation. It was hypothesized that because the second language would not be subject to such maturational restraints, the emergence of a second language would approximate more nearly to the theoretically hypothesized order of language acquisition. Of course, this is not the case because as the previous discussion has shown, second language development is subject to other influences.

The more mature psycholinguistic abilities of the second language learner seem to be among the factors which facilitate more rapid acquisition of the early stages of the second language. It seems that within a comparatively short time — i.e. 18–36 months — the emerging bilingual child can be functioning linguistically similarly to non second language peers. Some linguistic strategies may also be transferable to the second language from knowledge of a first language — e.g. the use of nouns/pronouns and word order. Others may be language-specific and require new rule acquisition — e.g. the formation of relative clauses or interrogatives.

To conclude, the theoretical framework for second language acquisition seems to derive mainly from that of first language. There are hypotheses about the acquisitional nature of the second language, which is influenced possibly more by affective variables and less by psycholinguistic factors than first language acquisition. The semantic and contextual features of input for the development of second language are hypothesized as being more influential than structural aspects which would agree with findings in first language development. However, there remains controversy over the efficacy of some selective, structured input where unstructured second language input may not be triggering appropriate second language development.

It is worth pointing out that most of the research previously done has looked mainly at aspects of syntax when investigating language acquisition. Future research could redress the balance by investigating different aspects of development — e.g. as semantic, pragmatic or phonological development — in second language acquisition (see Chapter 6). Furthermore, future research could investigate more varieties of bilingualism, taking into account more of the sociocultural aspects and patterns of language use which co-occur to make bilingualism heterogeneous. Some of the possible consequences of this heterogeneity are hypothesized, in the following section, in the notion of semilingualism.

SEMILINGUALISM

The concept of bilingualism which is developed in this book is one where the bilingual's linguistic repertoire is seen as functioning within an integrated, whole linguistic system. The different languages will have been acquired in different linguistic environments and they will function in different and complementary communicative contexts. Thus the linguistic repertoire of the bilingual may be similar to that of a monolingual in either language but will not be identical. In other words, the L1 of the bilingual speaker will not be similar to that of the L1 monolingual because she may have acquired a non-standard form or a contact-dialect. The L2 that has been acquired will not be identical to the language of a native speaker. For example, she will not use it in all the contexts that a native speaker would use it, and so the functions and vocabulary will differ. Finally, the L1 and the L2 of the bilingual speaker will not be the same structurally or pragmatically.

The uniqueness of the language profile offered by the bilingual speaker is fundamental to appreciating the concept of bilingualism. It has implications for the choice of standardization of populations for bilingual language assessments — possibly for all assessments of bilingual individuals. It has implications, too, for the clinical and pedagogic management of the bilingual child, for example, offering bilingual input in order to offer both languages an opportunity to enjoy mutual learning and communicative environments.

There is a position which argues that there is the 'ideal' bilingual, where the speaker has mastery of the two languages equal to a monolingual in each language; she is a 'bi-monolingual'. Anything less than this, as measured on tests (e.g. vocabulary, sentence construction and literacy) means that the speaker is, to varying degrees, **semilingual** (Skutnabb-Kangas, 1978).

The semilingual will not be a 'balanced' bilingual, that is, because of being an emerging bilingual, neither language will be acquired satisfactorily. As a result, concept development may not progress, the child will fail in the education system and compensatory education will be deemed necessary.

The means by which it is shown that there is monolingual mastery, or conversely, semilingualism, is by achieving on tests and assessments, such as Basic and Interpersonal Communicative Skills (BICS) and Cognitive and Academic Language Proficiency (CALP), devised by Cummins (1979). There are three controversies in this assessment which make it a dubious assessment tool for bilingual children, according to Martin-Jones and Romaine (1986). First, it is standardized on monolingual English speakers. Secondly, it is literacy based; indeed, Cummins notes the mis-match between low test scores and reported good oracy skills. Thirdly, and most seriously, the two parts of the test infer that surface structure competence means communicative competence and, in some ways, confuses semantic development with cognitive development. Thus failure on the surface structure implies failure of communicative competence, and failure to handle semantics implies retardation of cognitive development. A child may have problems in developing communicative competence and also cognitive concepts, but these difficulties may not be appropriately accessed or assessed through surface structure tests or semantic tests. It is recognized that the relationship between language/communication and language/cognition are complicated. So it may be more accurate, and serve the emerging bilingual child better, to draw the lines of this relationship less simplistically, acknowledging the restrictions of assessment tools; for example, non-verbal acultural assessment items may be an alternative. This debate is most important, not least because of the association that the semilingualism has with a 'deficit' theory.

Semilingualism — and associated terms such as **additive** and **subtractive bilingualism** — is a term which is gathering a great deal of support. 'Additive' refers to any positive effects on the L1 resulting from learning L2, while 'subtractive' means the converse (McLaughlin, 1978). Assessments, such as those cited above, lend a credibility to an idea which is not endorsed by other research findings. Day (1979) showed that nursery-age children who were Creole–English developing bilinguals acquired standard English as well as maintaining Creole English. Furthermore, a study in northern England among Bradford Panjabi-speaking schoolchildren (Rees and Fitzgerald, 1971), assessing the children on the Porch Index of Communicative Ability for Children (PICAC), showed that the mother tongue of these children was not adversely affected by the acquisition of English.

No one can be in doubt that education both in the established and the emerging language in the early years of formal education would be best for the developing bilingual child. The break from home to school would be less traumatic, and concept formation in both languages would benefit. Indeed, this is one of the motivating ideas behind the semilingualism school of thought. However, the implications of the semilingual idea are obvious in educational and clinical work. If certain forms of assessment procedures are employed then referral for remedial help may be a consequence, that is, remedial help in only one language and counselling for the giving up of one language (usually the non-school language and the language of the community), all of which is extremely controversial and possibly unnecessary if assessment tools appropriate to the bilingual population were used.

Children who have been assessed on their expressive language skills in both languages, and who show depressed profiles in comparison with their bilingual peers (Duncan and Gibbs, 1987),

34

are not semilingual. Rather they are potentially language handi-capped, with a language learning problem *per se*, and would demand more investigation from a speech therapist.

CONCLUSION

The issues involved in research related to bilingualism have been discussed in this chapter. The clinical and pedagogic implications of the findings have been noted throughout. The aim has been to show the importance of some language theories and the notions of language development they engender. It is these notions which underpin the work in clinical and educational establishments, thus affecting and shaping the lives of bilingual children. Practitioners cannot afford to be unaware of them in their work. It is hoped that further research will contribute to improving our understanding of bilingualism and its linguistic disabilities.

3

The Challenge of Working with Minority Languages

Jane Stokes and Deirdre M. Duncan

INTRODUCTION

Wherever the speech therapist/teacher/psychologist chooses to work, she is faced with the challenge of finding out about the community in which she works. This is particularly so when that community uses languages other than English. Communication disorders can only be distinguished from problems in learning English if the speech therapist has a sound knowledge of the socio-linguistic, cultural and historical context of the bi/multilingual population she is working with, and has access to linguistic information of the language(s).

This chapter describes various ways of tackling the challenge of working with speakers of minority languages by looking at the clinical and pedagogic implications of language demography and cultural background, giving some linguistic description of the two most spoken minority languages in the UK, and finally offering suggestions about setting up small-scale language research projects.

LANGUAGE DEMOGRAPHY

The first aim the practitioner involved with the bilingually language handicapped should set herself is to discover what languages are spoken within the geographical area for which she is responsible. Various sources can be consulted about the range of languages spoken in the UK; *The Other Languages of Britain* (1985), based on the work done by the Linguistic Minorities Project, is particularly recommended. Local information is available from borough councils, education authorities and community organizations. Smith (1982) examines the difficulties of obtaining reliable estimates of different populations of minority languages. This is primarily because, in the absence of any question on language in the national (British) Census, information about language is often based on birthplace and/or surnames on the electoral register.

Furthermore, there can be a reluctance on the part of some districts to collect information about the numbers and distribution of the bilingual communities in their area. This arises from the quasi-political nature of this information which is highly sensitive to misuse and negative interpretation. Yet this information is necessary for services working with bilingual communities if they are to be effective, particularly those working with bilingual children with special needs. These services can seek to equip themselves with appropriate language resources to meet the linguistic needs of their clients.

When information about the general language demography of the area is not available, the practitioner can collect specific information about the bilingual clients in their caseloads or in their classes which will be clinically and educationally helpful. This may sound obvious, but routine collection of statistics on language spoken does not seem to be standard practice in many speech therapy departments. In the UK it is not unusual to find practitioners who are unaware of the languages spoken by their clients and omit to record this information. It is to be hoped that such practices are a thing of the past. Within most services it is quite possible to incorporate into routine initial interviews questions about patterns of language use, which can be recorded as part of statistics collection and used to plan service delivery at a district level.

Implications

When appropriate questions are asked about the bilingual language handicapped caseload or class, useful information can be obtained for modifying and improving intervention and resources.

For example, information about the range of languages spoken by the children in the clinic/class, the geographical distribution in the neighbourhood and the relative proportions of the different languages will indicate the need for other language resources, their type and time allocation, and their placement. Chapter 7 discusses this in more detail. Clearly, gathering information about language distribution has implications for staffing levels, time management, liaison channels and management protocols for the bilingual child.

CULTURAL AND HISTORICAL BACKGROUND

In addition to information about languages spoken, the speech therapist needs to become acquainted with the cultural and historical backgrounds of the populations with whom she is working. This is for two reasons, as follows. First, with a broader perspective she can best modify her own cultural practices when she is familiar with the culture of her clients, and the history of the community to which the client belongs. For example, there are patterns similar to many immigrant bilingual groups, such as a migrant workforce gradually establishing itself into family and community networks, with tendencies to develop either socially self-sufficient communities wanting more linguistic autonomy, or becoming more integrated and monolingual.

Refugee groups will have a very different history of arrival and integration. In order to view the community in its historical and cultural context the practitioner will need access to information on patterns of migration, socioeconomic class, religion and age distribution. She will also need to understand something of employment patterns, housing conditions and educational facilities and to be aware of the effects of racism on the population.

The second reason why the practitioner should be familiar with the culture of the bilingual client's community has more direct implications on case management. For appropriate advice and management to be successful, the practitioner will need to have some knowledge of the family structure of the bilingual child's community; for example, whether the family is an extended or nuclear one, or whether there have been any adjustments made as a consequence of living in the UK. Further, she would be aware of the child-rearing practices of the community; for example the role of play, and the pattern of adult–child communication.

Finally, it is fundamentally important to see the individual client and her family within their cultural perspective, that is whether they are involved in maintaining their language and culture, or otherwise, and their personal circumstances regarding child-care and child-minding — is it the parents or others, and what are the patterns of language use of the primary caregivers? This kind of information is best acquired through contact with local community organizations, in the UK through the Commission for Racial Equality and by working alongside people from the linguistic minorities who can act as mediators of their culture and are an invaluable resource.

LINGUISTIC INFORMATION

Once the practitioner has some knowledge of the pattern of language use in the community with which she is working, she needs to collect information on the linguistic characteristics of the commonly spoken languages in that community. So, for example, if she discovers that Gujerati is widely spoken by the population, and that it is maintained as a home language by children at school in her district, she needs to do some research on the language. She will need to find out where in the world the language is spoken, what language group it belongs to and whether or not it is a written language. If possible, she should endeavour to find out about grammatical structure, word order and whether or not it is a highly inflected language (i.e. whether word endings are used to signify tense, number and gender). Information on this, and on phonology if available, will be important in the analysis of the child's first language and will help to orientate the practitioner. It may be possible to explain some irregularities in the child's language, or to predict developmental sequences, although this should be approached with caution. (Sources of information on different languages are given in the Bibliography.)

CHARACTERISTICS OF BENGALI AND PANJABI

As an example of the kind of information which would be useful to practitioners, we present some basic information on the characteristics of Bengali and Panjabi. The projects described in Chapters 4 and 5 deal with speakers of Bengali (Sylheti) and Panjabi. The speech therapists working on these projects collected this information in the course of their research. We would maintain that this type of information should form part of the resources available to any practitioner working with minority languages.

Language distribution

Bengali is, after English, the language spoken by most schoolchildren in London (ILEA Language Census, 1987). There are substantial numbers of Bengali speakers in many of the larger cities in the UK and also in smaller towns. The information collected in the 1987 ILEA Language Census indicates that numbers of schoolchildren speaking Bengali are likely to go on increasing because of the concentration in the younger age-groups.

Panjabi forms the largest linguistic minority in several London boroughs, and in cities such as Birmingham, Wolverhampton, Coventry, Manchester, Bradford, Huddersfield and Leeds. As with Bengali, there are substantial numbers of Panjabi speakers in the smaller towns.

Origins of speakers

The majority of Bengali speakers in the UK originate from Bangladesh (formerly East Pakistan). As is often the case with immigrant populations, large numbers of them come from a particular district. For example, the Bangladeshi communities come mainly from the Sylhet district which lies to the north-east of Dhaka, the capital. The Panjabi speakers in the UK come mainly from a geographical area in the north-west of the subcontinent, which covers three distinct political territories: the state of Panjab in India, its neighbouring area in Pakistan and the adjoining Mirpur district. Mirpur has a distinct dialect. A small number of Panjabi speakers in the UK come from East Africa, this group having emigrated from the Indian subcontinent at the turn of the century. In the UK there are also some Panjabi speakers from south Malaysia. A similar range of geographical origins pertains in many emigrant Panjabi speaking communities throughout the world — e.g. the USA, Canada and Australia; for further details the reader is referred to *The Other Languages of England* (Linguistic Minorities Project, 1985).

Language family

Both Bengali and Panjabi are Indo-European languages deriving from Sanskrit. The Indo-European family, as its name suggests, includes the major European languages, and Bengali and Panjabi have similarities with these. They share many grammatical features with other north Indian languages (e.g. Gujerati and Hindi), but differ from the Dravidian languages, spoken in southern India (e.g. Tamil and Malayalam). Bengali and Panjabi are distinct languages, not generally mutually intelligible, and with their own script. Sikh Panjabi speakers use the Gurmukhi script, and Muslim Panjabi speakers use Urdu script.

Word order

The basic word order in both Bengali and Panjabi is subject–object–verb (SOV). This compares with the subject–verb–object (SVO) order of English. So, for example:

the boy eats rice
S   V   O

would be translated in Bengali (Sylheti) as:

[pua bat khai]
boy rice eats
S   O   V

and in Panjabi as:

[munda tʃʰa| khaa]
boy   rice eats

The verb comes at the end of the sentence.

Adverbials (A) tend to precede the verb in both languages, in contrast to English; for example:

I am going out
S   V   A

would be translated in Panjabi as:

[me ba: dʒanda]
I   out   go
S   A   V

and in Bengali (Sylheti) as:

[ami bara dʒai]
I   out   go
S   A   V

Questions

In both Bengali and Panjabi, questions are formed either by intonation alone or by the insertion of a question particle, or question word, with no alteration of word order. Unlike English, there is no auxiliary 'do' and no inversion of the verb; for example:

What does the baby wear?

is translated in Bengali (Sylheti) as:

[beibi kita   phinda?]
baby what wears?

and is translated in Panjabi as:

[kaka ki   banda he?]
baby what   wears?

Negatives

Negatives are formed by the addition of a negative particle, in Panjabi before the verb, and in Bengali (Sylheti) after it; for example:

This is not mine

is translated in Bengali (Sylheti) as:

[eta amar na]
this mine not

and is translated in Panjabi as:

[e   mera naii (ai)]
this mine not (is)

Note that in both languages the copula 'to be' can be omitted; this is another feature of Panjabi and Bengali. In English the auxiliary 'do/does' is inserted in the formation of the negative but there is no equivalent in Bengali (Sylheti) or Panjabi; for example:

The child does not speak

is translated in Bengali (Sylheti) as:

[batʃa mate na]
child speaks not

and is translated in Panjabi as:

[bʌtʃʰa bolda naii]
child speaks not

Postpositions

These correspond to prepositions in English and, as the term implies, come after the noun phrase. They occur in Bengali (Sylheti) and Panjabi; for example:

in the cupboard

is translated in Bengali (Sylheti) as:

[kuborder bitre]
cupboard inside

and is translated in Panjabi as:

[kubord vitʃ]
cupboard in

Determiners

Determiners are used, but less frequently than in English as there is no equivalent of definite or indefinite articles, although numerical words are sometimes used as articles. Demonstratives (this, that, etc.), possessives (my, his, etc.) and quantifiers (some, many, etc.) are used.

Compound verbs

These are commonly used in Bengali (Sylheti) and Panjabi. They are similar to phrasal verbs (e.g. 'to go shopping') or particle verbs

43

(e.g. 'to make do with') in English, with the main semantic weight being borne by the lexical verb, usually in its root form. The second verb, sometimes termed the formant verb, often changes its original meaning and modifies the main verb. Common formant verbs include 'to go', 'to take' and 'to give' in both Bengali (Sylheti) and Panjabi.

Pronouns

There are first-, second- and third-person pronouns in Bengali (Sylheti) and Panjabi. The third-person pronoun has no gender distinction — i.e. the same word is used for 'he' and 'she'. The form of the second person varies according to the relationship with the speaker — i.e. formal or informal.

The information provided here has concentrated on Panjabi and Bengali (Sylheti), and this should give some indication of the type of grammatical information it would be useful for the practitioner to collect when working with minority languages. More detail on the characteristics of north Indian languages can be found in Jackson's chapter (in Abudarham, 1987; see also Mobbs, 1982, and Tolstaya, 1981).

RESEARCH PROJECTS

Once information on specific languages and the communities who speak them has been collected, speech therapists will need to develop research projects to look at aspects of assessments and remediation with bilingual clients, just as they do for other groups of clients. There is an urgent need to develop criteria-referenced language assessment procedures, and it is on these that we focus in the next chapters. However, it is equally important to discuss and test out different methods of therapy. With the appointment of bilingual co-workers, the decision as to which language should be used becomes a real choice in therapy.

Practitioners need to consider whether offering intervention only in English is in fact the most effective way of working with a client. Therapy in a child's first language may have a corresponding effect on a child's second language, but as yet we have no firm data to support this (see Chapters 9 and 11).

Rukshana, a 4-year-old Bengali (Sylheti) speaking child was attending a language unit where the only language used was English. She was showing delay in both English and Bengali (Sylheti) and progress over three months of therapy in English was slow. A Bengali (Sylheti) speaking assistant started to work with her, under supervision of a speech therapist, daily for a period of two months. Working entirely through Bengali (Sylheti), the assistant helped her to expand vocabulary and increase the range of syntax and semantics she was able to express. The corresponding improvement in her English abilities and her general confidence allowed her to transfer out of the language unit after three months.

Similar projects need to be tried on a larger scale in order to see if this is a general pattern; in order to base our assessment and remediation on sound theoretical ground we need information on stages of normal language development, phonological processes in minority languages, non-verbal behaviour, and so on. Only once we have started to accumulate data on normal speech and language development in minority languages can we begin to judge whether a child is showing delay or disorder. Once it has been decided that a project should be set up in a minority language community, the following factors need careful consideration.

Aim

The area of investigation needs to be defined. The practitioner should decide, for example, what the main focus should be (syntax, phonology, pragmatics or semantics). This decision may be based not only on the particular interest of the practitioner, but also on the types of referral that are received. The patterns of occurrence of certain pathologies may also affect this decision. So, if, for example, it seems that there are significant numbers of dysfluent children within a particular language community, it would be appropriate to investigate. If Yoruba is a language widely spoken in a particular area (this African language has an increasing number of speakers in ILEA schools according to the 1987 Language Census), the speech therapy service may decide to investigate it. However, it is not enough to decide to look at Yoruba; within a language it is important to define the particular aspect of investigation. Stages of normal language development in minority languages may be an area for investigation, as in the projects described in Chapters 4 and 5. Alternatively, the development of meaning in second language (L2) English in L1 speakers of minority languages may be the focus of research, as in Chapter 6. Constraints, such as time, finance and access to computers, will obviously play a part in the decision as to what to research.

Methodology

Methodological details need consideration. Numbers of subjects, age range, research design, statistics and data sampling techiques will vary, depending on the focus of the research. For example, if a practitioner decides to look at development of phonology, a longitudinal study may be most appropriate. If she is more interested in the incidence of voice disorders, then a cross-sectional design would be more relevant.

The three projects described in the following chapters have similar designs: 24–30 subjects, over an age range of 18–60 months, and divided by six-month intervals into 4–5 groups of six children; this constitutes a cross-sectional design. The Panjabi project also has a longitudinal component where some subjects are followed over a long period of time. All the projects observed the subjects in naturalistic settings. If the investigation is looking at language comprehension, an experimental setting might be more appropriate, so that stimuli can be carefully controlled. For some projects matched subjects may be needed, involving statistical calculation, while for others single case studies may be more relevant. Information may also be gathered on sociolinguistic patterns through the use of questionnaires.

If the practitioner can attach herself to an academic institution, then she will be able to seek advice and support on these matters from a supervisor and other academic staff. It may also be a precondition of funding that the practitioner should register for a higher degree.

Resources

Once the need for a project has been identified, it will be necessary to obtain the support of local managers. This is best done by presenting the need for the work in terms of the implications for service delivery in time and efficiency. For example, if it has been decided to look at attitudes to communication aids in a particular community, the researcher will need to show that the information on this will improve the service to this client group. If it had been found that communication aids are issued but not used by this community, then a survey of attitudes towards communication aids would have financial implications as it may well be that inappropriate aids were being issued.

Important considerations in planning a project include the provision of a room to work in, with access to appropriate facilities (telephone, computer and photocopier), provision of stationery, travel expenses, and audio or video tape recording equipment of the right quality. The researcher will need to consider if other staff are required to work on the project; such as clerical assistants, research assistants and speakers of the minority language being investigated. The researcher also needs to decide the status of any bilingual staff employed: are they to be used as interpreters, or will they be expected to undertake data collection and transcription; devise questionnaires and analyse language data? Appropriate salaries will need to be provided.

It is important to make good links with the minority community to be researched, and to obtain the trust and approval from local community organizations. The researcher may decide that a joint project with other health or education workers would be most useful — and will therefore need to liaise with health visitors, psychologists and teaching or nursing staff, as necessary. If the researcher is registered at an academic institution, she will have access to library facilities, and advice on research, and will need to have a supervisor with relevant interests. If the research is clinical, it will be important to choose a supervisor with some clinical experience, if possible.

Once all these resources have been considered, the researcher will need to prepare a detailed protocol to apply for funding. Possible funding sources need to be investigated. Health and education authorities have some research monies, and details of these are obtainable from local offices throughout the UK. If the work is to be undertaken together with people from another profession, joint funding may be available — i.e. funding shared between health and education, or health and social services. In the UK charitable institutions which provide funding are listed in the *Charities Directory* and *A Guide to Grant-Making Trusts* which are available in libraries. The Centre for Information on Language

Teaching (CILT), in London, publishes a useful directory of sources of funding. The King's Fund, based in London, considers applications from health service workers and provides useful advice on writing protocols. Similar funding bodies and directories exist outside the UK and practitioners considering research should investigate them thoroughly if seeking their support.

Problems

It is worth knowing the problems that may arise when setting up a research project. Obvious problems surround the acquiring of sufficient money; some funding agencies may specify that they only provide money for certain areas of work (e.g. unemployed people). There may be problems in the scale of the project: it is often the case that an initial idea for research has to be considerably refined, so that the project can concentrate on a much smaller area than at first envisaged.

There may be problems liaising with the minority community, who may be wary of white monolingual researchers doing work in their community. It is essential to obtain the trust and co-operation of local community leaders to ensure that the community understands and endorses the investigation. Linguistic minorities are understandably cautious of how the results of any research project could be interpreted and used.

The most appropriate research will come from a need identified by the linguistic minority themselves. If, for example, there have been inappropriate referrals to speech therapy because of inadequate assessment procedures, it is clear that research into appropriate assessment procedures will help to alleviate the problem.

The results obtained from the research may be difficult to interpret, and the data obtained may be less useful than originally planned. However, there may be 'spin-offs' from the study which had not been anticipated. Dissemination of the results of the project will need careful consideration, so that findings can be used in the most constructive way.

CONCLUSION

In this chapter we have presented a possible model for the setting up of a research project, and considered the aims, methodology and resources needed. We have also examined the practical aspects of working with minority languages, which we firmly believe to be not a 'problem' area, but a challenge. We have used Bengali (Sylheti) and Panjabi as examples, but we hope that practitioners working with other minority languages will be able to draw some advice from this chapter on how to tackle working in the field. Following on from the suggestions made here, we present in Chapters 4–6 examples of how three different speech therapy services identified the need for, and undertook, research into minority languages.

4

First Language Panjabi Development

Nita Madhani

In Newham the clinical medical officers were concerned about the Asian children who were not performing on the two-and-a-half year developmental language screen (Barnett and Fletcher-Wood, 1981; Barnett, 1983). The high percentage of uncompleted screens led to two queries:

1. Are the children not performing on the screen because of inadequate exposure to English?
2. If there is a genuine primary language delay, how can the Asian children be screened and offered appropriate intervention?

The screening procedure in English highlighted the difficulties of assessing the language development of the high proportion of non-English speaking children. Direct translations of this screen into another language would not tap the equivalent linguistic structures (see Chapter 8). Enquiries to India and Pakistan concerning Panjabi acquisition failed to provide any normative data.

In 1984 a research grant was funded by the North East Thames Regional Health Authority (NETHRA Sangmed fund) to allow investigation into the acquisition of Panjabi. The ILEA 1981 Language Census indicated that Panjabi was the most widely spoken minority language in Newham.

The aim of the research was to establish a linguistic profile of the developmental stages of Panjabi speaking children. This profile would provide a yardstick to screen and assess a child's language development and also offer guidelines to clinicians and teachers for appropriate intervention, should there be a primary language delay.

SUBJECTS

Consent was obtained for children to be selected from local child health clinics across the borough. Criteria for selection were based on the children not having any known hearing problems, physical defects or abnormal birth history. The primary language had to be Panjabi and the children must have been born in England. The two Panjabi groups, Muslims and Sikhs, were equally represented in a mixed-gender sample. Socioeconomic class distinctions were not considered as the division would have to be made by English class structures, the appropriateness of which is debatable.

DESIGN

Forty-eight children had been selected to the above criteria; 24 children were included in the project, and the extra numbers allowed for any potential drop-outs during the span of the project. Each child was followed up at six-month intervals. There were four groups and the sample size increased at each age level, thus:

6 children at 18 months   —   group 1
12 children at 2 years   —   group 2 (groups 1 + 2)
18 children at 2½ years   —   group 3 (groups 1, 2 + 3)
24 children at 3 years   —   group 4 (groups 1, 2, 3 + 4)

This produced a longitudinal language data of Panjabi over a two-year period.

PROCEDURE

All children were seen in the home environment by a bilingual speech therapist (English–Panjabi). Each family received two initial visits from the speech therapist and a further two visits at six-monthly intervals. The initial visit was intended to meet the parents of the children participating in the project, and to explain

51

the reason for and procedure of the project. A child information sheet (Fig. 4.1) was completed by the parents and the child was assessed on a simple non-verbal matching task which increased in complexity. This task was based on the English norms of non-verbal behaviour (Cooper, Moodley and Reynell, 1978).

Subsequent visits resulted in recording language in the home environment. At each stage in the project, 100 child utterances were recorded and analysed. All the utterances analysed occurred in child–mother (or siblings) interactions. A basket of toys, which had stacking, mechanical and symbolic play toys, was provided by the experimenter.

Figure 4.1 Child data sheet

NAME: M. F.

D.O.B.

C.A.

DATE: PLAYGROUP:

FAMILY HISTORY

Siblings   ....

Ages of children   ....

Order of the subject in family   ....

Father's occupation   ....

Mother's occupation   ....

Parents' country of origin   ....

Any known speech or language impairment in the
family   ....

Language spoken at home   ....

PERFORMANCE ON THE NON-VERBAL TASKS:

1. Demonstrate symbolic use of objects   ....

2. Ability to object/object match   ....

3. Ability to object/picture match   ....

4. Ability to picture/picture match   ....

ANALYSIS

By its nature, the study was intended to be descriptive in order to furnish the lacking information. The analysis of the data was based on LARSP (Language, Assessment, Remediation and Screening Procedure; in Crystal, Garman and Fletcher, 1976) profile which attempts to summarize the most frequently occurring elements in a child's language at certain ages. The Panjabi data are not profiled on the original LARSP form, but the principles of profiling and tabulating the data were applied in the same manner as in LARSP. Clause structure, phrase structure and word inflections were analysed into the first three stages, I–III, then tabulated according to age, and the number of elements present in the child's utterance. Stage IV marks the complex elements and does not always have the equivalent number of elements; complexities that occur beyond stage IV will not be discussed in this chapter (Table 4.1).

The clause structure consists of the main elements of an utterance: subject (S), object (O), verb (V), complement (C), adverbial (A) and question word (Q). The phrase structure consists of elements which modify the items in the clause structure: postpositions (Post), determiners (D), adjectives (Adj), verb particles (V-part) and compound verbs (VV). The word category marked the noun cases, tenses and plurals.

The order of elements in each stage are congruent with word order in Panjabi. For the purposes of this chapter, the data and analysis form only a part of the total study.

RESULTS

The results were charted in tabular form (Table 4.2) for each child. Stage I utterances are not divided into clause and phrase elements as they are single-word utterances.

Table 4.1 Clause and phrase structures across stages I–IV

	Clause structure	Phrase structure
Stage I	single words (nouns, verbs, other)	
Stage II	2 elements	2 elements
Stage III	3 elements	3 elements
Stage IV	4 elements	complex elements

Table 4.2 Record chart for subject's L1 Panjabi utterances

Stage I (0–1.6 years)	Stage II (1.6–2.0 years)	Stage III (2.0–2.6 years)	Stage IV (2.6–3.0 years)
Clause level			
Nouns (N)	SV	SOV	SOVA
Verbs	OV	SAV	SCVA
Other	SC/O	SCV	SOQV
	AX	AOV	
	QX		
	Neg x	XQy	tag Q?
Phrase level			
	NN	DNPost	
	DN	D Adj N	CX
	AdjN	Part-V	
	V aux	VV aux	
	VV	Eng-V	
	Pron	Neg-V	
	Cop		
	NPost		
Word level			
Tense markers, noun cases, plurals			

Stage I

Nouns

The nouns used at this stage were those which were most meaningful in the child's life. The nouns used were both Panjabi and English. Out of the 63 noun labels used at this stage, 39 nouns were English labels. Of the other 24 nouns, 8 were kinship terms, some of which do not have common English equivalents. The kinship terms reflect the effect of growing up in an extended family environment where adults other than the parents share the same household. The specific kin terms are easy to articulate and have sounds which a child would have acquired by 18 months. Most kinship terms have a consonant–vowel–consonant–vowel pattern. Anthony Carter (1984), in his study on children's usage of kinship terms, suggests that children learn the rules of addressing others by active learning as opposed to passive imitation. Adults would use different terms among themselves, but children are taught the correct terms for appropriate relatives; it is seen as a sign of respect and bonding between particular adults and the children. The English nouns used by children at 18 months were:

Toys — ball, teddy, car, bike, dolly
Food — coke, juice, jam, bread, crisps, ice-cream, sweet,
    biscuit, orange, apple
Household — telly, table, phone, video, photo, carpet, sofa,
    settee
Other — cartoon, shopping

Panjabi kinship terms were:

Grandfather — [baba]	Grandmother — [bibi]
Paternal uncle — [chacha]	Paternal aunt by marriage — [chichi]
Maternal uncle — [mama]	Maternal aunt by marriage — [mami]
Maternal aunt — [masi]	Paternal aunt — [phuphi]

Verbs

The verbs used at this stage were those that expressed the child's immediate needs. All the verbs were in root form, that is without any tense or gender markings. The verbs used were [de] — to give; [pi] — to drink; [dekh] — to look; and [le] — to take.

Table 4.3 L1 Panjabi subjects(S)–verb(V) combinations at 2 years

	S	V
Panjabi	Babu	aja
Gender	masc	V(masc)
English	Babu	come
Panjabi	Rani	aji
Gender	fem	V(fem)
English	Rani	come

Table 4.4 L1 Panjabi objects(O)–verb(V) combinations at 2 years

	O	V
Panjabi	apple	khana
Gender	masc	V(masc)
English	apple	eat
Panjabi	roti	khani
Gender	fem	V(fem)
English	dinner	eat

In stage I there were many vocative utterances to attract attention — for example [mama dex] — mummy look. There were also stereotypical phrases such as Panjabi greetings, 'Bye-bye', 'Oh no' or jingles like 'Happy birthday to you'.

Stage II

Clause level

Children at 18 months were using some two-word utterances, but they were not frequently used. At 2 years most of the utterances had two elements which were either subject–verb (Table 4.3) or object–verb (Table 4.4) combinations. All the two-word utterances indicate that children mark the subject–verb concord right from the start. (In Panjabi the verb inflection has to agree with the gender of the noun which would be masculine (masc) or feminine (fem).) 'Rani' and 'roti' are of feminine gender and take the feminine verb marker, whereas 'Babu' and 'apple' are of masculine gender and take the appropriate masculine verb marker.

Question forms used at this stage were: [ki] — 'what', and [kithe] — 'where'. The construction of Panjabi is simple and the question word is inserted before the verb, for example:

What is — [ki he]
Where is — [kithe he]

Negation

At 18 months and 2 years the children signalled negation with nouns, verbs and other words; it is used to mark straightforward refusal. In Panjabi negation is marked by adding the negative particle [nei] before the verb, for example:

Panjabi	English	Analysis
[nei lena]	no take	neg. verb
[nei bar]	no outside	neg. adverb of place
[nei book]	no book	neg. noun

Phrase level

The data of the 2-year-olds indicate a marked increase in the use of the phrasal elements. At this stage the categories that appear include: determiner noun (DN), adjective noun (Adj-N), noun-

noun (NN), copula and the auxiliary form of the verb 'to be' — [hona], compound verbs (VV), pronouns (Pron) and postpositions (N-post). Compared to the English stage II phrase level, the Panjabi stage II phrase level appears to have the auxiliary and copula verb and the pronoun categories established.

The only determiners used at this stage are: [e] — 'this', and [meri] — 'my'. The adjectives used were 'big' and 'small', and both of them were marked for gender (in agreement with the noun).

Verbs

The verbs are marked for present tense and gender. The auxiliary verb is not marked consistently at this stage, but all the children in the data used it in their utterances at some stage. The verbs used by all the children at stage II were: [hona] — 'to be'; [lena] — 'to take'; [pana] — 'to put'; [kheldna] — 'to play'; [dena] — 'to give'; [dekhna] — 'to look'; [pina] — 'to drink'; [ana] — 'to come'; [jana] — 'to go'; [khana] — 'to eat'.

Compound verbs were formed using the verbs [lena], [dena] and [jana]. The copula was used most frequently with a complement, for example: [dolly he] — 'is dolly' (CV in Panjabi).

Pronouns

The pronoun category was the most heavily used category at stage II. Demonstrative pronouns [e] — 'this' and [au] — 'that' were used, and the first-person pronoun [me] — 'I'.

Postpositions

All the children signalled 'in' — [vitʃ], 'on' — [te] and 'to' — [nv] by the age of 2 years, for example: [bæg vitʃ] — 'bag in', meaning 'in the bag'.

Stages III and IV

Clause level

The clause structure at stages III and IV indicated that the children use more complex utterances which have three or more elements. Their vocabulary is greater and they also master the prosodic rules to use language in a creative way, for example, altering the intonation of an utterance to convert it to a question; and SOV, SCV and SAV structures are used by all the children. There are different constructions of SOV and SAV utterances, but the most common SCV construction is [æ *'noun'* hæ], meaning 'this is *"noun"'*, where a noun is used with the copula verb [hona] — 'to be'. The number of three-word elements used are less compared to the two-word utterances, that is O/CV. In Panjabi, O/CV utterance is accepted as a mature form of utterance.

At stage IV the only structures used by all the children were SOAV and SAQV. Some children start to use the tag question (tag Q) — [hena], which is the equivalent of 'isn't it'. It is the only form of tag question used in Panjabi.

Phrase level

The DNPost and D Adj N categories were not widely used at these stages. The pronouns signalled were: [me] — 'I'; [tu] — 'you'; [usi] — 'we'; [e] — 'this'; and [au] — 'that'. The auxiliary verb was used appropriately and consistently with single verbs; and with compound verbs, they were just beginning to emerge in some children, as indicated in Table 4.5.

The new postposition used here was [nal] — 'with'. At the stage IV phrase level there were no specific changes, with some children using the connector [te] — 'and'.

Word level

The present tense markers [di/da] (M/F) were used consistently from the age of 2 years. Plurals were only signalled for the nouns. At 2 years the noun cases used were genetive case [da/di] (M/F), to mark possession. The case ending must agree with that of the noun, for example: [daddy di book] — 'daddy's book'; 'book' is feminine and thus [di] is used.

Table 4.5: Auxiliary verb and main verb usage at stages III–IV in L1 Panjabi development

usi	bar	chul gaje si	(Panjabi)	'we had gone out' (English)
S	A	V	(Clause III)	
Pron	Post	VV aux	(Phrase III)	

CONCLUSION

The children's developmental language profile suggests that Panjabi clause structure development shares similarities with English clause structure development. However, the phrase structure and the word level develop in a different manner. For example, in Panjabi the negative verb (Neg-V) formation occurs early since it is the only mature way to express negation. At stage II the negative particle [nei] was used in an immature way with all the elements of the clause structure, but from stage III onwards the negative particle was only used with verbs, which is the mature form. Another novel feature at stage III phrase level is the use of English verbs as verb particles with another Panjabi verb — e.g. [kick marna] is the equivalent of 'to kick' in Panjabi, but if translated into English, it becomes 'kick to do'. This has been marked as Eng-V at the stage III phrase level. It can also be marked as an English–Panjabi compound verb.

At all stages, more than 50% of the nouns used were given English labels. Children use the English labels since they are used in the home environment; many of the children would not know the Panjabi labels for these nouns. There are differences in the pronunciations of the English words. Children who have not mastered the phonological rules of English often generalize the phonological rules of Panjabi and apply them to English words — e.g. /pʰen/ becomes [pen] and /kʰʌp/ becomes [kʌp]. Another example is when a schwa vowel is inserted between the consonants in clusters — e.g. /spvn/ becomes [səpvn]. Lexical borrowing is a further example of generalization of linguistic rules across the two languages — e.g. 'books' become [bvkā], where the English lexical noun is retained with the Panjabi plural inflection added.

The information obtained from this project will be used to design a language screen in Panjabi, for Panjabi speaking children up to the age of 3 years. The non-verbal tasks used in the project indicate that the matching concepts seem to be acquired in a similar way to English speaking children. The non-verbal tasks provide useful clinical information for Panjabi speaking children and should form a part of the early language developmental screens.

5

First Language Bengali Development

Jane Stokes

The impetus to embark on a study of Bengali language development arose from a desperate clinical need felt by speech therapists
working in Whitechapel, East London. In this part of London
there is a population of approximately 20 000 Bangladeshi people
who maintain Bengali, or rather a regional variety of the language,
Sylheti, as their dominant language.

SYLHETI

The majority of Bangladeshi people living in Whitechapel originate
from Sylhet, a region north-east of Dhaka, the capital. They speak
a regional variety of standard Bengali, known as **Sylheti**. Since
migration to London, a strong awareness of the linguistic identity
of these speakers has developed (Smith, 1985). Many feel it is
misguided to treat Bengali and Sylheti as a single linguistic entity.
There is as yet no detailed description of Sylheti, which differs
from standard Bengali in several respects; syntax and lexicon are
distinctive, as is phonology. It was only during the course of the
work carried out in Whitechapel that the extent of the differences
between standard Bengali and Sylheti emerged. Major aspects of
structure are common to both, as outlined above: the subject is not
always explicitly stated, as it can be inferred from the verb ending;
and the formation of tenses is different for some verbs, and there
are some major lexical differences in pronouns, postpositions and
adverbials. In phonological terms, aspiration is distinctive in
standard Bengali, but this does not appear to be so in Sylheti. This

study did not set out to examine the differences between standard Bengali and Sylheti, but there is a need for a detailed investigation of these.

Sylheti is not a written language, although there is some evidence that in the past there was a written form of the language. Differing views exist on whether standard Bengali and Sylheti are mutually intelligible; in general, it seems that Sylheti speakers can understand standard Bengali, but that Bengali speakers unfamiliar with Sylheti have some difficulty in understanding it. There is a strong feeling in Whitechapel that Sylheti should be regarded as a language in its own right. This has led to an insistence that Sylheti speakers be appointed to work as community workers and interpreters. Certainly, the children in Whitechapel are exposed to Sylheti almost exclusively and speak it at home. Within Sylheti there are some small regional differences, mostly in phonology and lexicon, between speakers coming from different districts within Sylhet.

Despite the lack of detailed knowledge on the development of Bengali, and its relation to the regional variety Sylheti, it was felt important by the speech therapists in Whitechapel to develop some means of assessing the language abilities of the Bengali (Sylheti) speaking children referred to speech therapy.

THE WHITECHAPEL PROJECT

Some 30% of referrals to speech therapy in Whitechapel are from children under age 5 who have had no exposure to English. Therefore, there was a very real need to develop an assessment procedure for the detection of language delay in Bengali (Sylheti). In order to do this, information on the normal stages of language development was necessary. It seems that neither in Bangladesh nor in India is the field of developmental psycholinguistics very widely researched. It did not prove possible to obtain any study of the developmental stages of Bengali in India or Bangladesh.

A project was therefore set up in 1984, funded by the King's Fund in London, to investigate the stages of language development in normally developing children speaking Bengali (Sylheti) in Whitechapel. It was decided to concentrate on the children under five years, as this is the population from which the majority of speech therapy referrals come. The project employed a speech therapist working half-time over three years, and a Bengali (Sylheti) speaking assistant working half-time over eighteen months.

In order to collect information about children's language development, it was decided to concentrate on their expressive language. This was felt to be a more direct reflection of a child's language abilities than would be their abilities in comprehension.

A comprehension test is less revealing about a child's actual language competence than a profile of expressive language. A comprehension test requires more structured intervention on the part of the person administering it, and it was felt to be more important to obtain a sample of speech in as natural a setting as possible. This was best done by recording expressive language at home. In this context it is difficult to exclude gestural and situational cues, so that it would be difficult to get an accurate assessment of comprehension abilities.

It was necessary to develop a method of analysis of the child's expressive language. The most useful format seemed to be a profile such as that used widely by speech therapists in the UK, the Language Assessment Remediation and Screening Procedure (LARSP) (Crystal, Fletcher and Garman, 1976). This is used to obtain information about a child's syntactic abilities. It gives an indication of the normal order of acquisition of different syntactic structures. These are divided into stages based on number and complexity of elements in an utterance which correspond loosely to age levels.

In recent years there has been a shift away from looking at syntax in isolation. It is clear that syntax does not develop in the abstract, but depends on meaning relations and vocabulary acquisition. It was felt that it was important to investigate these areas of language development alongside the development of syntax.

A framework for analysing the semantic and lexical abilities of the child was necessary. In the development of a profile of syntactic, semantic and lexical abilities it was inevitable that English was taken as a starting-point, given the lack of information on Bengali (Sylheti) language development. However, as the project progressed, more language-specific information emerged and corresponding adaptations to the framework for analysis were made.

The language of 30 children between the ages of 18 months and 4 years was recorded. Information on the language development at these ages was felt to be most useful to speech therapists. The children were divided into six-month age bands: 18 months to 2 years, 2 years to $2^{1}/_{2}$ years, $2^{1}/_{2}$ to 3 years, 3 to $3^{1}/_{2}$ years and $3^{1}/_{2}$ to 4 years. Six children, three boys and three girls, were seen at each age level. These children were selected randomly from health visitors' records. All had passed various developmental checks, and neither they nor their siblings had any history of hearing loss or any other disability. All children were exposed only to Bengali (Sylheti) at home, and the majority were born in England and had not spent any time in Bangladesh.

The children were visited at home three times for a period of $1^{1}/_{2}$ hours each; a minimum of 200 utterances was collected, by audio tape recording and by transcription at the time by the research assistant. There was no attempt to structure the recording session or to interfere with the normal interaction in the family. Apart from the inevitable effect of having a stranger in the house, the language was felt to be as natural and representative of the child's abilities as possible.

The framework for analysing the language covers the sentence syntax, semantics and lexicon of the child's expressive language. All utterances are analysed, including the responses to adult questions (these are excluded from analysis in LARSP). Children's responses provide useful information on their ability to converse, and on how they pick up what is said to them. Exact repetitions are discounted — i.e. where children imitate exactly what is said to them, without using any additional words and maintaining the same word order. Utterances which are incomplete or do not make any sense in the context are not analysed for syntax, but may be analysed for semantics and lexicon if appropriate.

While the framework for analysis has similarities with LARSP and the Profile in Semantics (Prism) (Crystal, 1982), there are differences. Some categories have been omitted because they did not seem to provide any useful information. Others have been adapted to suit the nature of Bengali.

The language of each child is analysed according to the framework and then compared with the language of the other children of the same age range. At each age features which are common to all children have been noted. Those features which appear to be typical of each age range, and which are not evident at the previous age range have been termed the **key features**. Therefore, each age range has certain characteristic features which mark it as separate in syntactic and semantic terms, and to a lesser extent, in lexical terms. It is hoped that this will aid the speech therapist in the analysis of the children's language. There should be no need to analyse every utterance, but instead the speech therapist can look for the key features typical of the age range of the child. It is also likely that if these key features are not apparent in the child's spontaneous language, there may be an element of language delay in Bengali (Sylheti).

Syntactic analysis

The syntactic analysis was loosely based on the LARSP categories. Some alterations were necessary to accommodate the differences in Bengali (Sylheti) structure. The stages used in LARSP correlate with ages; in this analysis stages are not used. The age bands act as stages, and the framework for analysis is organized on a scale of progressively longer and more complex sentence structure. The major one-, two-, three- and four-word utterances are recorded with information as to clause level and phrase level; VV, in the analysis, refers to a common construction in Bengali (Sylheti) where two verbs are used together in a way similar to the English phrasal verb (e.g. 'to go shopping'). Other structures are broadly similar to English. The framework for syntactic analysis is as follows:

Q	question word
N	noun
V	verb
ADV	adverb
ADJ	adjective
SV	
SO/C	complement (C)
O/CV	
S ADV	
V ADV	
NEG x	negative plus one other element
Q x	
VV	compound verb, made up of two verbs
ADJ N	
DET N	determiner
N POST	noun plus postposition
SC/OV	

SAV
C/OAV
AAV
NEG x y
Q x y
D ADJ N
SC/OAV
AASV
AAOV
NEG x y z
Q x y z
c x   connective
x c x

As can be seen, we are interested in the major syntactic structures. 'Yes' and 'no' responses are not analysed, nor are simple vocatives or social greetings, or calls for attention. As we are more interested in the early stages of language development, the more complex utterances are not analysed but note is made of them separately.

Differences between Bengali (Sylheti) and English may affect the pattern of use of some syntactic structures. As has been pointed out, the subject may not be explicitly stated in Bengali (Sylheti). For instance, OV may be a complete utterance in Bengali (Sylheti), which it would not be in English, and in Bengali (Sylheti) a determiner is not obligatory in most contexts; the determiner is used mostly for emphasis; and in the majority of sentences nouns do not require a determiner. Information which may be conveyed at phrase level in English may be conveyed, in Bengali (Sylheti), at word level. For example, the prepositional phrase 'at school' in English would be translated as 'school*o*' in Bengali (Sylheti). This would not show up in the syntax analysis, but in the lexicon analysis (see later).

The 200 utterances collected from each child were analysed according to this syntactic framework. From this analysis can be seen where the bulk of utterances lie and what are the commonly used structures and the gaps in a child's syntactic knowledge.

Children were grouped according to age level, and their use of different syntactic structures was compared. Syntactic structures which were used by all children at any age level were grouped as typical of that age level. The different age levels were then compared. Any structure which was present at one age level, but did not occur at the previous age level, was termed a key feature. Each level, then, had a series of key features — syntactic features which could be seen as typical of that age level in these children (see Results).

Semantic analysis

It was decided to look only at the semantics of the one- and two-element utterances. At the stage where a child is using simple syntactic forms it is interesting to see which meaning relations are being expressed, and what the developmental stages of sentence semantics are. At the three- and four-element stage the semantics are more predictable from the range of syntax and lexicon. Therefore, it was felt that to analyse the three- and four-element utterances for semantics would duplicate the information obtained in the syntactic and lexical analysis. The major semantic categories for analysis of the one- and two-element utterances are taken from Brown (1973) and PRISM (Crystal, 1982), and partly from Bloom and Lahey (1978). The categories used in the semantic analysis are as follows:

Agent: *bringing about the event, animate or inanimate*
Object: *affected by the event, animate or inanimate*
Goal: *person or place which is the goal of the agent or object*
Agent + object
Instrument: *used to perform an action*
Source: *person or place which is the source or origin of the agent or object*
Attribution: *specifies a characteristic or property of an object or person*
Change of location
Negation
Possession
Change of possession

Further semantic information emerges in the lexical analysis, for example, on verbs, which are crucial in the expression of different meaning relations. In the semantic analysis we are interested in the one- and two-element utterances. By analysing these we are trying to see which meaning relations exist when the syntax is not well developed. One- and two-element utterances will occur throughout the different age levels, but there will be proportionally more at the younger age levels.

In the same way as for the syntactic analysis, the language samples were analysed (one- and two-word utterances only) and the semantic categories used by all children in an age-group were identified. Any semantic category which occurred in the samples of all children within an age-group was termed a key feature of that age-group.

Lexical analysis

The analysis of the lexicon complements the syntactic and semantic analyses, and should be viewed alongside them. Additional semantic and syntactic information will emerge from the analysis of the lexicon.

Information on the lexicon was collected according to a framework devised to include all the major lexical fields. The range of words used in each major syntactic category was investigated, along with the morphology of nouns and verbs. The categories included in the analysis were as follows:

Nouns
    common
    proper
    family
Pronouns
Noun endings (plural, definite, subject, object, possessive,
              locative)
Verbs
    agentive (where an event, location, possession, state or
           change in these is brought about by an agent)
    agentive locative
    agentive possessive
    agentive state
    non-agentive (an event with no agent)
    compound verbs
Adverbs (time, manner, place)
Adjectives (colour, temperature, size, other)
Postposition (temporal, spatial, instrumental, manner)

Question words
tag
what [ki]
who [ke]
where [kunano]
why [kiare]
how [kila]
whose [kar]

Against each category, examples were recorded, but the number of instances of occurrence of each word was not recorded, that is the type, not the token. Children were compared across and within age levels, and some broad generalizations were possible. Key features could be identified in the morphology, but because of a wide variation in the actual words used by each child, it was not possible to pick out key features in the lexical fields.

Results of the syntactic and semantic analysis

A great deal of information was obtained as a result of the analysis. Information about the syntax and the semantics is best summarized by a list of the key features. From Tables 5.1 and 5.2 the speech therapist can see which features of syntax and semantics were used by all children in each age group; asterisked features refer to those which appear for the first time at that age. There is a steady progression through the ages in terms of length and complexity. For the most part, features which appear at one age then appear consistently in the older age-groups. There are a few exceptions to this (Adj, Neg x y z and SC/OAV). This may well be because of the variations in use of the children, and may be a fault of using relatively small numbers of children at each age. For the purposes of assessment these should be assumed to exist at the older age levels above that at which they first appear. The same is true for 'Goal' in the semantic analysis which appears for the first time at age 2–2½, but not at the 2½–3 level. However, as it appeared in the samples of five of the six children seen at this age, it can be assumed that it is widely used at this age.

Results of the lexical analysis

A summary of the results of the lexical analysis is given below. (More detailed information is available from the author on

Table 5.1: Key features of syntax

1½–2	2–2½	2½–3	3–3½	3½–4
N	N	N	N	Q
				N
V	V	V	V	V
Adv	Adv		Adv	Adv
	Adj*			Adj
SV	SV	SV	SV	SV
SO/C	SO/C	SO/C	SO/C	SO/C
O/CV	O/CV	O/CV	O/CV	OC/V
	Adv x*	Adv x	Adv x	Adv x
Neg x	Neg x	Neg x	Neg x	Neg x
				Q x*
		VV*	VV	VV
			AdjN*	AdjN
	DetN*	DetN	DetN	DetN
		NPost*	NPost	NPost
		SC/OV*	SC/OV	SC/OV
		SAV*	SAV	SAV
			C/OAV*	CO/AV
	Neg x y*	Neg x y	Neg x y	Neg x y
				Q x y*
			SC/OAV*	
		Neg x y z*		Neg × y z
				Q x y z

Table 5.2: Key features of semantics

1½–2	2–2½	2½–3	3–3½	3½–4
Agent	Agent	Agent	Agent	Agent
Object	Object	Object	Object	Object
	Goal*		Goal	Goal
	Attribution*	Attribution	Attribution	Attribution
Change of loc.				
	Change of loc.	Change of loc.	Change of loc.	Change of loc.
Negation	Negation	Negation	Negation	Negation
	Possession	Possession	Possession	Possession
Ch. of Poss.	Ch. of poss.	Ch. of poss.	Ch. of poss.	Ch. of poss.

request.) As we have already stated, key features could be identified in relation to morphology and they are presented in Tables 5.3 and 5.4.

It was not possible to identify verb endings used by *all* the children in each age-group, as there was considerable variation in the tenses used. Table 5.4 shows the endings used by four out of six children in each age-group.

Table 5.3: Noun endings

Years:	1½–2	2–2½	2½–3	3–3½	3½–4
	-r poss	-r poss	-r poss	-r poss	-r poss
	-o loc	-o loc	-o loc	-o loc	-o loc
		-e subject*	-e subject	-e subject	-e subject
		-re object*	-re object	-re object	-re object
				-o loc*	-o loc

Note: Asterisked items occur for the first time at that age.

Table 5.4: Verb endings

1½–2 years
-i   simple present
-si   simple past
-tam   future, implying 'want to'

2–2½
-i   simple present
-si   simple past
-tam   future, implying 'want to'
-bo }
-mu }   future

2½–3
-i   simple present
-iya   continuous present
-si   simple past
-lam   perfect
-tam   future, implying 'want to'
-bo }
-mu }   future
-le   conditional

There was no change at the 3–3½-year level and the 3½–4-year level. The children used the same range of verb endings as at 2½–3 years. Information on the other lexical categories analysed can be summarized as follows.

Nouns

There is a steady increase in the number and range of nouns used as the child gets older. Words for food are acquired early and used widely.

Family names

A wide range of these is used by all children. In Bengali (Sylheti) different terms are used to describe, for example, a paternal uncle and a maternal uncle. Some of these family names are acquired before age 2.

Pronouns

A variety of pronouns meaning 'that one' are used from an early age. The distinction between formal and informal pronouns is acquired after $3^{1}/_{2}$ years (Bengali (Sylheti) makes a distinction between second- and third-person formal and informal).

Verbs

There is a steady increase in the number and range of verbs used across the age-groups. Compound verbs are used widely from $2^{1}/_{2}$ years.

Adverbs

Adverbs of place are most commonly used. Adverbs of time are only used after $3^{1}/_{2}$ years.

Postpositions

These are not used much until after $2^{1}/_{2}$ years. There are more examples of spatial postpositions than of any other type, and a wide range is used.

Adjectives

Adjectives of size and quality (good, bad) develop earliest. Colour adjectives are not used much until after 3 years.

Question words

There is a steady development of these related to semantic complexity. Words for 'where' and 'why' develop at around 3 years and 'who' at the $3^{1}/_{2}$–4-year age level. Question words relating to time begin to be used by some children at the $3^1/_2$–4-year age level.

English words used commonly by the children

A number of English words occur in the output of the children studied. Some of these words have been adopted by the Bangladeshi community as a result of English influence (e.g. 'light'). Some are used in the absence of an alternative Bengali (Sylheti) word and would be used by people in Bangladesh (e.g. 'table'). The majority of English words used are nouns; there are a few exceptions to this (e.g. 'under', 'cooking', 'shooting'). Some English words are pronounced differently (e.g. 'pram' is pronounced 'ferem'). There does not appear to be a correlation between the frequency of use of English words and having siblings who attend school. Some of the children who show the most instances of English words have no siblings at school. There is probably a wide range of attitudes within families towards the adoption of English words and the usage of the parents may affect the child's use. Here is a list of the commonly used English words, in order of frequency of use:

> sweet
> baby
> cartoon
> ball
> doll/dolly
> plane
> bread
> cycle
> bike
> dog
> frock
> film
> photo
> English (= English person)
> bath

There is a slight increase in use in the older age-groups, but the proportion of English words used does not change with age.

Use of the assessment procedure

It is hoped that the information obtained on the language develop-ment of Bengali (Sylheti) speaking children will help speech therapists to analyse the expressive language of these children, and thereby make some assessment of their abilities in syntax, seman-tics and lexicon. On this basis some judgement should be possible as to whether a child's language is developing along normal lines.

In order to use the assessment procedure, a sample of Bengali (Sylheti) language should be obtained containing a minimum of 50 utterances. This should preferably be obtained at the child's home and in as naturalistic a setting as possible. It may be necessary to allow $1\frac{1}{2}$ hours for this, in order to overcome shyness on the part of the child and to ensure that the language is representative. A Bengali (Sylheti) speaker will be necessary to assist in the record-ing, transcription and analysis, and it is obviously important that he or she is trained in the necessary skills.

The sample should be transcribed, but each utterance need not be fully analysed. The sample should be scanned for the key features of the age level at which the child is — e.g. a child of 2.3 would fall in the age-group $2-2\frac{1}{2}$. The key features of this age-group are shown in Table 5.3, and particular note should be made of the asterisked features which appear for the first time at this age. It is important to establish whether the child's language shows any of these key features. In addition, the information on lexicon should be used to see whether the children are using the range of lexicon typical of their age-group.

If children are found not to be using several of the key features of their age-group, further investigation may be necessary. The speech therapist might need to elicit certain structures to see if the child is able to use them, if they have not occurred in the sample of spon-taneous language. If it is evident that the child's language is more typical of a child in a younger age-group, it can be tentatively assumed that the child's language is delayed in Bengali (Sylheti).

Clearly, as the sample of children seen in this project was small, with only six children at each age, the key features cannot be viewed as norms. However, they do serve as examples of language used at each age, and as such should provide speech therapists with an invaluable guide as to what can be expected. Further research is needed to replicate these findings, and to extend the assessment procedure.

An example of analysis

Below an example of analysis is given to show how each utterance was examined in detail for syntactic, semantic and lexical content.

Child of 2.8

	SYNT	SEM	LEX
marsi	V		Agentive verb
I hit (past)			-si past
. (it : implied)			
puk gasegi	SV	Agent	Noun
the insect went away		Change of loc.	-si past (gi = filler)
gorom na	Neg x	Attribution	Adj. temp.
(it's) not hot	Adj	Negation	
thænda na	Neg x	Attribution	Adj. temp.
(it's) not cold	Adj	Negation	
ou daho	OV	Object	Agentive verb
look at that			Pronoun -o present

6

Aspects of the Development of Second Language English

Deirdre M. Duncan

INTRODUCTION

Much of the second language English research focuses on the syntactic aspects of language development. The purpose of this chapter is to attempt to redress the balance by looking at some semantic and sociolinguistic features of second language (L2) English. The chapter will describe a study investigating the development of these features in the emerging L2 English of Panjabi and Bengali pre-schoolers, and some clinical and educational implications are drawn.

BACKGROUND

The study is set in the UK's second largest city, Birmingham, which has a population of about 1 million, with many ethnic minority communities. For various reasons, there is a lack of detailed information about the language demography of the city. Despite this, it is clear that in the west of Birmingham — where this study is based — the largest ethnolinguistic communities are Panjabi and Bengali (Sylheti). Consequently, the study chose to look at these communities.

It is worth pointing out that minority (particulary language minority) communities are quite distinctly and separately located within a district (Linguistic Minorities Project, 1985). The language minority population distribution has implications for educational and clinical service delivery. It should be possible, with appropriate information collection, to target provision of language resources to particular areas and thus to maximize the benefits of the service.

It is important to understand that these communities are maintaining their linguistic and cultural heritage, so that second- and third-generation children are growing up to be bilingual in their community language and English. All those working with bilingual children, particularly speech therapists, face the challenge of assessing, teaching and remediating children for whom there are no adequate developmental guidelines. In second-language English development it is not acceptable to use norms and age stage information which pertain to monolingual English children (see Chapter 8). Specific information about bilingual language development is essential and crucial. Chapters 4 and 5 have furnished information on mother-tongue development, and this chapter aims to supply information on the emergence of L2 English.

THE PROJECT

In the mid-1980s the speech therapy department in the West Birmingham Health Authority obtained funding from a governmental body called the Inner City Partnership (ICP) to support linguistic research with the bilingual population in the district. The original proposal was to investigate bilingual language development in the pre-school population, concentrating on the Panjabi and Bengali communities, as mentioned above. For numerous reasons, the proposal had to be modified to become an investigation of L2 English development. It is hoped that future research in the UK will study other community languages such as Gujerati or Vietnamese.

Aims

The aims of the project to be discussed here were as follows:

1. To investigate the semantic aspects of second language English acquisition, namely semantic relations, lexis and function;

RESULTS

2. To obtain sociolinguistic information which would be useful for clinical and educational purposes.

METHODOLOGY

The L2 English population group studied is Panjabi and Bengali pre-school children — i.e. under-5s. The data was collected from four age-groups: 3, 3.6, 4, and 4.6 years over a period of six months (October–March). Data samples were collected from a different subject from each age-group in the two language groups on alternate months. Thus there were twelve subjects for each language, and six subject cells in each age-group. Due to some subjects dropping out for various reasons — e.g. non-cooperation; illness and moving out of the area — certain subjects were sampled twice.

The subjects were controlled for age and time in nursery. They all had older siblings attending school, and normal hearing and medical development; and they all spoke Panjabi or Bengali in their homes. There could be no tight control for socioeconomic factors, and although all the subjects came from nursery schools within a 1-mile radius, there may well have been differences in financial and educational background. Gender was not included as a criterion, yet the proportion fell almost equally; and parental permission was obtained. Confirming normal non-verbal cognitive functioning was done by the Goodenough 'Draw a man' test (the controversies of which are acknowledged), observation and teacher report.

RESULTS

Linguistic semantics is to do with how words — lexemes — relate to the world outside (i.e. reference) and to themselves (i.e. structural semantics). The investigation of the development of reference occupies much of the literature on the semantics of emerging first language, for example, the **Semantic Feature Hypothesis** (Clark, 1973), semantic field emergence, and semantic mismatch. However, in second language acquisition, one would expect reference to be largely established. So the development of second language semantics would mainly focus on those aspects of

77

structural semantics to do with grammatical meaning relations, and to a lesser extent, on lexical references — although this would depend on the age of the second language learner. Structural semantics has two aspects: lexical and grammatical. The lexicon is analysed along paradigmatic relations of sameness, inclusiveness, opposition and dissimilarity, and syntagmatic relations of collocation, that is word predictability. Grammatical semantics — semantax — analyses the meaning relations of grammatical participants in a sentence.

There is very little detailed descriptive data about the development of these aspects in first language, so the second language data will be presented here, structurally analysed and comparisons made with first language development where possible.

Lexicon

Semantic Fields

It is clear that lexical inventories (i.e. word lists) on their own can divulge little about the internal lexical organization of developing child language. It is this internal organization which reveals the salient features which the child is learning. Procedures such as Profile in Semantics–Lexicon (Prism-L) (Crystal, 1982) offer a categorization scheme which reflects ideas of salience and semantic fields. A version of the procedure is presented (Table 6.1), modified to accommodate the data, which analyses the lexes of the youngest group.

The first observation which can be made about this lexical information is that in a range of nearly a hundred items there are only fourteen which are common to more than half of the subjects in the group. Of these fourteen items, six are in the category 'people'. 'Teacher', 'boy' and 'girl' can be expected in the classroom vocabulary, while 'mummy', 'daddy' and 'baby' are more unusual, and may possibly be explained by these items being 'borrowed' from English by their Panjabi and Bengali repertoires. In the range of nine categories, only six have shared lexis. If the items 'bike' and 'car' were moved from the semantic field of 'vehicles' to that of 'toys', since they were used in both contexts, then there would only be five semantic fields sharing lexis. It should be noted that 'toys' is a questionable semantic field and children may prefer to categorize them in their 'real-life' fields (Crystal, 1987).

Table 6.1: Vocabulary items of the 3–3½ years age-group

Category	Item	No. subjects used item	Category	Item	No. subjects used item
People	mummy	4	Clothes	boot	3
	daddy	4		shoe	2
	baby	3		coat	2
	boy	4		sock(s)	2
	girl	4		hat	1
	teacher	3		trousers	1
	friend	1		T-shirt	1
	postman	1		shirt	1
	lady	1		button	1
	men/man	2	Food	cake	3
	gingerbreadman	1		ice cream	2
	doctor	1		biscuits	1
	policeman/police	2		sweet(ie)	1
Vehicles	bike	4		bread	1
	car	5		apple	1
	trucks	1		Coca Cola	1
	policecar	2		rice	1
	fire-engine	1	House	(electric)light	2
	tractor	1		bed	2
	train	2		door	1
	bus	2		toilet	1
	boat	2		carpet	1
	scooter	1		seat	1
	airplane	2		house	1
	motor-bikes	1		garage	1
	rocket	1		swing	1
Toys	doll	3	Utensils	cup	2
	ball	2		basket	1
	book	2		knife	1
	camera	1	Animals	dog/doggie	4
	gun	1		fish	3
	robot	1		spider	3
	pencil	1		cat, horse, cow, bird, chicken, goat, lion, monkey, snake	2
	balloons	1		(guinea)pig, rabbit, fox, frog, donkey, sheep, lamb, tortoise, mouse/mice, ducks, butterfly, dragon, crocodile, tiger, camel, elephant, giraffe	1
	ring	1			
Body	face	1			
	ears	1			
	leg	1			

The semantic field of animal names shows the most inter-subject variability. Apart from 'dog', 'fish' and 'spider', there are 26 items which are shared by only one or two subjects. This most probably reflects a classroom influence where there are many didactic materials involving animals. Not included in Table 6.1 are the attributive features for this age-group which cover a range of four categories: *size* — big, little/baby; *quantity* — all, a lot of/lots of, some; *colours*; and *numbers* — particularly 'two'. The latter two fields clearly reflect a classroom influence on the second language development. The attributive features are a noticeable area of growth in the language development of the older age-groups (3–4.6 years). There are few developmental indicators in lexical acquisition, yet in first language it is suggested that facial lexis (e.g. eyes, nose) is among the earliest emerging. This suggestion does not find much support in this second language sample.

Overextension

There is only limited evidence of overextended vocabulary use in the second language data, as was predicted (Rescorla and Okuda, 1984). For example, the unknown referent 'worm' was called 'snake', and 'ostrich' was called 'duck'. A further explanation of limited semantic mismatch was that when subjects did not know a particular referent which they realized was conceptually distinct, they simply admitted the fact by saying 'I dunno'. There is one idiosyncratic example where one subject used the item 'guinea-pig' to refer to an ordinary pig. He was a Bengali Muslim, and it is possible that for religious reasons he may not have wished to use the word 'pig', and he would have been familiar with the word 'guinea-pig' because there was such an animal in his nursery classroom.

Similarly, the notion of **semantic fuzziness** (Rosch, 1973) is not supported by the data of the second languge learners. There are few labels referring to 'stereotypes', and ample illustration (e.g. the animal category) of non-stereotypical labels which are associated with later development.

Paradigmatic relations

The following are some examples from within-subject data of these sense relations.

Synonomy — bike = motor-bike

little = baby
police = policeman
Hyponomy — no superordinates found in the data for this
age-group, only subordinates
Opposition — big / little
robot / lady robot
Non-binary contrasts — number, shape, colour.

Semantic relations (Semantax)

In first language studies much of the research is on the semantics
of two-word utterances (Howe, 1981) because this is recognized as
the usual starting-point for grammatical development. The
youngest subjects in this study all had second language utterances
at and beyond the two-word level. The semantic relations in this
age-group are quite developed and could be seen to develop more
in the older age-groups.

The following semantic relations were already established in the
repertoires of *all* the subjects in the age-group 3–3.6 years:

Actor Dynamic — e.g. boy dance
Dynamic Goal — e.g. made this car
Actor Dynamic Goal — e.g. I do this one
Experiencer Stative Goal — e.g. I got a big one car
Experiencer Stative Goal — e.g. I want it

The semantic specifications which are established are:

Definiteness — e.g. this car
Attribution — e.g. look at *big* car, *two* men
Possession — e.g. *my* bike
Location — e.g. *on* bike

The following semantic relations feature in *some* subjects' data:

Dative — e.g. give me garage
Experiencer Stative Locative — e.g. her sleeping in bed
Actor Dynamic Goal Locative — e.g. he putting fish in his house
Temporal — e.g. now look, come on then

Other aspects of semantax will be summarily presented as follows:

Interrogatives feature in the data of only two subjects: one used 'who', 'what' and 'where', and another used only 'what'. Other interrogatives, such as 'which' and 'why', appear in the speech of the older subjects. This is in line with information from first language studies.

Negatives are used by all the subjects to mean non-existence (e.g. 'no shoes'), refusal (e.g. 'a scooter no'), denial (e.g. 'no lady robots'), as well as in the more sophisticated syntactic forms (e.g. 'can't', 'didn't', 'haven't'), which are more established in the older subjects.

Pronominal reference shows a clear developmental pattern. Self-reference is established in the data of all the youngest subjects (e.g. 'I', 'me', 'my', 'mine'). The non-self-referent 'it' is also emerging. The occurrence of 'you' and other referents are signalled in some of the data. The older subjects' data reflect a clearly different pattern, where all the referents have a similar distribution, although gender referencing may not be fully established.

Situation types (i.e. verb meanings) fall into two groups: dynamic and stative. **Dynamic situation** types basically describe the subject's action, and **stative situation** types basically describe the subject's qualities and state of being (Quirk et al., 1985). The distribution of situation types in the youngest subjects' data show the following three aspects of development. First, the most frequently occurring verb meanings across all the subjects were semantically non-specific. They are: 'look', 'look at', 'go', 'put', 'see', 'got', 'finish', 'do'/'doing', 'be'('am', ''s', 'is'), 'want'/'wanna' and 'give'. Secondly, the most common after these in all the subjects' data are dynamic situation types such as 'dance' and 'ride'. Thirdly, stative situation types occur the least frequently — i.e. in only two subjects' data. They are: 'like', 'know' and '(be) sleeping'. The data of the older subjects sees a growth of both dynamic and stative meanings, which seems to reflect their context dependence. This developmental pattern in verb meaning acquisition seems to follow that noted in first language development.

As a footnote, one subject was noted to use 'am' for 'have' (e.g. 'I am this gun' and 'I am the book'). It is a good illustration of the potential for idiosyncratic development within the broad

constraints of language acquisition (Yoshida, 1978).
Simple relations were reflected only in the data of this age-group. There were no utterances containing compound meanings, such as contingency or probability, although these might have been present in the mother tongue. The older subjects' data suggest that compound meanings were developing (e.g. contingency, 'if').

FUNCTIONS

The intentions of the child's utterances have been analysed by Halliday (1973) in seven categories of language function:

Instrumental — the 'I want' function
Regulatory — the 'do as I tell you' function
Interactional — the 'getting along with others' function
Personal — the 'here I come' function
Heuristic — the 'tell me why' function
Imaginative — the 'let's pretend' function
Representational — the 'I've got something to tell you' function

There may be a developmental aspect to these functions, with instrumental being the earliest to emerge in first language English and representational being a function mainly used by adults.

In the data of the youngest subjects the following pattern emerges instrumental is clearly established in the data of this age-group. Regulatory (e.g. 'shut up', 'stop') is developing, and interactional (e.g. 'you go in there', 'wait for me') is emerging. It could be that the little evidence of these functions is associated with the limited interaction with peers in English, and with the absence of non self-referents, which was noted in the previous analysis.

The representational function is well established in the data of all the subjects. This suggests a different pattern of development from first language English, and there could be several explanations. It could be that the informal routine with the investigator actually promoted this category of response, or it may be that the school environment generally encourages the child to express propositions. It has been noted that this function is most common in adult speech (Halliday, 1973), so it could be that the subjects were influenced by this model in their second language learning.

Heuristic function seems to be present only in the data of two subjects. Overall, the subjects do not seem to use second language English as a medium for learning, exploring or problem-solving.

Only one example of the personal function can be found in the data for this age-group ('I like it'). The absence of other expressions of feelings or attitudes could be for many reasons, and possibly requires a degree of confidence and intimacy not established by this age-group. It may also be associated with the sparcity of stative verb meanings at this stage, which usually carry the meanings to express these sentiments.

There are no examples of the imaginative function. Symbolic noise from one subject is the only approximant. It is interesting that the sampling did not capture this function. Further, when the investigator suggested 'pretend' situations, the subjects always responded in the 'here and now'. It seems that this function may not emerge until later in second language development.

There are obvious implications from the functional analysis for the interaction between the monolingual adult clinician and the emerging bilingual child. The practitioner might aim to assess which language functions the child uses in each language, bearing in mind that in the early stages of L2 English development, certain language functions may be preferred (e.g. instrumental) by the child, while others may not (e.g. imaginative).

SOCIOLINGUISTIC FINDINGS

Supplementary to the above investigation the patterns of language use by the subjects were noted. The three aspects of language use discussed here concern: exposure to second language English; some factors which seem to influence language choice; and affective variables.

Exposure to L2 English

The range of second language ability in the subjects could not immediately be explained by age or exposure to English in the nursery. So it seems that L2 English input from siblings, even in homes where parents did not encourage English, is a most influential factor.

Language-orienting factors

Despite being in an English environment, the subjects exercise language preferences and some of the factors influencing this choice have been noted. When playing in the **play-house** in the classroom, subjects, regardless of age, usually chose to speak in their mother tongue. This could possibly be due to the strong association between the home atmosphere and the first language. **Private talk** with a close companion, almost regardless of age, was usually conducted in the mother tongue. Across age there seems to be a move away from using mother tongue in school. The investigator noted that the **close proximity of an adult English speaker** may be sufficient stimulus to cause the subject to change from mother tongue to English while speaking to a companion.

Affective variables

It was clear that the personalities of the subjects influenced their second language acquisition, that is, the loquacious and the quiet. The effects were illustrated by the different strategies the subjects adopted towards second language acquisition — e.g. 'join in when you can', or a more reserved attitude.

DISCUSSION

Chapter 2 has put forward some hypotheses about the development of second language English. The results of the semantic analyses of this study will be discussed with reference to these hypotheses and some framework for interpretation offered. Bearing in mind that the hypotheses were developed on the basis of syntactic, not semantic acquisition, the 'fit' will not be exact, but may offer some guidelines.

The Natural Order Hypothesis

Given that there is very little information on the natural acquisition order of semantics aspects of first language English, it seems that second language English has some similarities, and many unique patterns of semantic development.

The Input Hypothesis

Here the premiss is that second language develops from 'comprehensible input'. This study has shown that there seem to be many sources of influential input for the second language learner, and aspects of the development of lexis and function seem to be affected by classroom input. The second language input from siblings and home would need further investigation.

The Affective Filter Hypothesis

The variation of second language abilities among the subjects goes some way to supporting this idea. More support comes from the subjects who could not be included in the study because, despite similarities in age, exposure to second language English and normal functioning, they had low performance skills in English manifested by non-cooperation and timidity.

The Monitor Hypothesis

There does not seem to be much support for this hypothesis from the data of the youngest group of subjects, possibly because of the meta-linguistic awareness which seems to be involved in this hypothesis. There are examples of false starts, hesitations, and so on, but there do not seem to be any clear examples where these relate only to semantic aspects.

The Acquisition–Learning Hypothesis

Evidence supporting this hypothesis would come from examples of lexis, or semantic relations which challenge the meaning and selection criteria of the item(s) in first langue English usage. For example, some features of verb meanings may be developmentally constrained and emerge later, such as intentionality, as in the contrasts 'fall'/'drop', 'see'/'watch' and 'say'/'tell'. Thus examples of non-target language use may not appear until a later age. There do not seem to be examples of non-target semantic use of this kind in the data of the youngest subjects, but there may be some in the data of older subjects.

The data and analysis presented here suggest that the development of semantic aspects of second language could offer many insights about the theoretical nature of language acquisition as well as yielding helpful clinical information.

PART TWO

Management, Assessment and Therapy

7

Working with Interpreters

Sarah Barnett

It is ironic that in speech therapy, concerned with communication disorders, the problems posed by language barriers have yet to be overcome. These barriers are particularly complex for the speech therapist, for apart from the obvious communication barriers, there are also the difficulties she finds in examining the nature of the disorder itself, let alone those of alleviating it.

This chapter is concerned with how speech therapists can work with interpreters, but first we will look at the need for bilingual staff in speech therapy, models of bilingual service provision in other agencies and then examine the nature of interpreting. A future model of trained and employed bilingual facilitators is discussed in the latter part of the chapter.

THE NEED FOR BILINGUAL STAFF

Working in districts where many referrals are from families with whom the therapist does not share a language makes discussing their case history, analysing the disorder or providing suitable therapy virtually impossible. The speech therapist is left with feelings of inadequacy about the unprofessional level of service she can provide, and the client and family do not receive the help they need. This unsatisfactory situation is increasing in its frequency.

The employment of bilingual staff is clearly essential, but the seemingly obvious solution of employing ethnic minority speech therapists who speak the local languages is difficult for three reasons. First, in some districts linguistic diversity is such that there are more languages spoken than there are posts covering the variety of speech therapy specialisms; secondly, there are as yet very few ethnic minority speech therapists; and thirdly, they do not all necessarily wish to specialize in communication impairment within one community. A possible parallel development to seeking ethnolinguistic speech therapists would be the employment of bilingual facilitators, that is bilingual people trained and employed to collaborate with speech therapists and, perhaps, other related professionals such as psychologists.

There are controversial issues surrounding the employment of interpreters in the public services. Some people are of the opinion that employing interpreters would mask the need for bilingual staff within each profession and therefore block the drive for training ethnic minority people. Similarly, it is felt that working with an interpreter reflects the racism operating in society, in that in such situations there is a 'black recipient' and a 'black mouthpiece' but (usually) a 'white authority' person. Meanwhile there are those members of British society — including taxpayers — who are unable to gain access to services due to the persistent communication barrier.

When a child or adult is referred for speech therapy, the stages of case-history taking, assessment and therapy are involved. Where the client is from a (potentially) bilingual environment, it is often necessary to enlist assistance from someone who can speak the other language(s) concerned.

The communication process

In the case-history taking of a potentially bilingual child, whose parents and therapist do not share a common language, there is an obvious communication barrier. Attempts to communicate via gesture and mime, dictionaries and drawing may be made. However, it is generally a frustrating experience for all concerned, being effortful, embarrassing, time-consuming and unproductive. It is not possible to take an adequate case history in this way.

Further, a detailed case history is arguably more important in the investigation of a bilingual child's communication in view of the scarcity of language assessment instruments — monolingual or bilingual, standardized or otherwise — in languages other than English. It is necessary to enquire about the family's pattern of language use (i.e. who speaks what, to whom and when), the communicative purposes each language has had for the child and also the duration and type of exposure the child has had to each language. Without this basic data, more specific linguistic symptom collations cannot be placed in context, which is necessary for their interpretation. Thus assistance from one who can speak the relevant languages is essential in the case-history taking.

This language barrier to communication similarly affects the processes of advice-giving, treatment option discussions, progress discussions, and so on. Written communication is also impeded, with appointments, letters, advice leaflets and reports which need to be translated.

The diagnostic process

In the assessment of a child's communication skills, despite the current lack of useful tools, the principles in the bilingual context remain the same as those for the monolingual English child. The therapist will be investigating the child's language(s) both receptively and expressively with respect to form, content and use (Bloom and Lahey, 1978).

For the therapist investigating skills in a language she does not speak, there is a clear necessity for assistance from someone who does speak the language(s) concerned, both in administering receptive tasks and in eliciting and recording samples of speech and language for linguistic analysis.

The therapeutic process

Following the history taking and assessment of the child's skills an intervention strategy is usually necessary. This again will often require assistance from a speaker of the relevant language(s) in its implementation; in the advice and counselling of the parents of a pre-school stutterer, for example, or in the direct implementation of a language programme in the child's mother tongue. Thus it can be seen that at all stages of management of a bilingual speech therapy client there is a need for assistance from one who can speak the appropriate language.

Other agencies have difficulty with only the first point above, the communication process. Let us look at the strategies they have used to overcome this difficulty.

MODELS OF BILINGUAL SERVICE PROVISION

Over the course of time different agencies, with their differing needs and access to resources, have developed various models in crossing language barriers. The status, training, role definition and renumeration for the bilingual people engaged in these varies considerably

The interpreting continuum
Translators
Conference interpreters
Community interpreters
Community workers
Link workers
Advocates
Bilingual workers
Family and friends
Children

The **translation** of the written form from one language to another is highly skilled professional work. The training for this work is at graduate level, and there is specialisation according to the type of work translated — from poetry to computer programming manuals to academic texts on Marxism; the professional body is the Translators' Guild.

Conference interpreters are also highly trained, again at graduate level. The languages in which training is offered tend to be European, which enjoy relatively high status in Britain and the western world.

Community interpreters, in contrast, have considerably lower status, primarily reflected in their poor pay. As yet there is little opportunity for training. The Institute of Linguists' Community Interpreters Project has established an excellent training model in Cambridgeshire (Corsellis, 1988). Two pilot training projects have been set up by the London Interpreting Project (LIP) in Wandsworth and Camden (LIP, 1985). Elsewhere training, if any, has been limited to a seminar on the role of the community interpreter, but little else (Shackman, 1983). It is felt (Corsellis, 1986) that the skills required in community interpreting are in fact greater than those in conference interpreting for three reasons. First, in conference interpreting one is usually concerned with the standard dialectal form of the two languages involved, and with the formal register of each, whereas in community interpreting there is likely to be a much wider variation of dialectal forms to contend with, plus the full range of registers to cross. Secondly, in conference interpreting the more demanding emotional and/or confrontational types of dialogue are likely to be encountered far less frequently than they are in community interpreting. Thirdly, in conference interpreting there is some specialization, but within community interpreting this has yet to be established. The Institute of Linguists' Project has insisted upon training modules specific to types of agency — e.g. 'Police, courts and probation work' or 'education welfare, social services and local government. However, in most community interpreting agencies one is covering a vast variety of organizations and professions with their specialisms, jargon and networks.

The roles of the **community worker** and community interpreter have been blurred, particularly where a bilingual community worker has been asked to act as an interpreter. A community worker is likely to be working on behalf of their client. A community interpreter should remain impartial with their duty being towards the communication process. In the health service two specific models of bilingual service provision for ante-natal care and childbirth have been developed.

The **link worker** scheme, initially funded by the Department of Health and Social Security (DHSS), has been developed by the Asian Mother and Baby Campaign. These workers are bilingual and have nursing training background. As the name suggests, they are employed to 'link' between the mother and the midwife/hospital staff/health visitor.

The **Multi-Ethnic Women's Health Project** (1985) financed by the Kings' Fund has been developed by City and Hackney's Community Health Council (East London). This scheme employs bicultural, bilingual patient-advocates who have personal experience of childbirth. The scheme is designed such that the consumer's interests remain paramount; the project's steering committee has strong representation from community groups. The advocates are not employed by the health authority, as it is felt that if they were part of the authority or arguably institutionalized racism, there would be a conflict of interests as for whose benefit they were working. Both these models are concerned with childbirth, the selection criteria requiring previous experience either as a practitioner or as a recipient of maternity services. Both models become extended into child assessment centre work. Arguments against the schemes run along the lines that the recipients may be done a disservice as the health professionals have less involvement with their patients, being more reliant on verbal reports from less medically qualified staff. One counter-argument to this is that professionals may be guarding their knowledge territory too jealously. Both models are successful and have much to commend them. However, there is a need for adaptation from primary health-care language needs to the more complex communication requirements of speech therapy and psychology (clinical, educational and psychotherapeutic). In the mid-1980s working in districts which had bilingual service provision was still the exception rather than the rule. Most clients and health workers either struggled on alone or used bilingual workers, family and friends or children. Despite their limitations, this is likely to remain the status quo for the foreseeable future.

Using other **bilingual workers** as interpreters varies in productiveness, according to factors such as language matching, bilingual skills, time availability, similarity of professional type of work and status, interpersonal skills, expectations of one another's role in this situation, dialectal variations and attitudes to dialects of different status. It should be appreciated that asking a bilingual health worker (e.g. a health visitor) to assist in a case-history taking means she has to take time out of her own workload that she will need to catch up on later. This extra time and work tends to go unrecognized and is not paid for, yet the person this is being requested of is often in a double-bind situation, feeling they have little option to say no.

Family and friends may be brought to the session by the client. The advantages here may be that the family already has a rapport with this person and aspects of confidentiality can be clarified between them. Possible disadvantages are that this person's skills in the therapist's language may be greater than those of the client, but not necessarily broad enough to place full confidence in the outcome of the initial speech therapy consultation. Further, it may be that the relationship between spouses, for example, where one speaks the therapist's language and the other does not may mean that one parent is excluded from discussion of their child. Indications as to the differential diagnosis between, for example, elective mutism and language delay can be missed in this way.

Finally, there are **children** often used as 'interpreters' for the family. This places a heavy burden of responsibility on one who cannot be expected to translate routine questions such as birth details. It can also cause role conflict between parent and child, and it frequently necessitates the 'interpreter' child missing valuable schooltime.

Apart from conference interpreters, the above models include little, if any, training in interpreting. Some discussion is given to the role of the interpreter *vis-à-vis* the client and the agency worker, but none is given to the skills needed in the art of interpreting.

The need for this training is not appreciated because the complexity of interpreting skills is generally unrecognized. The reasons for this are twofold. First, the heterogeneous nature of bilingualism is ill-understood — e.g. that there will be functional differences between two languages for most bilingual people. Secondly, the extent of differences between two languages and their conceptual and structural formats, leaving aside cultural variations, can render direct interpretation/translation impossible. This lack of understanding of the nature of bilingualism and the variation in linguistic forms leads to non-appreciation of the skills involved in interpreting. Consequently, there is a lack of recognition of the need for training in these skills which, in turn, leads to unreal expectations of lay bilingual people as interpreters.

Moreover, the pressures on a bilingual person to interpret on demand are often not recognized. Think of having to interpret, without preparation and for total strangers, a consultation about distressing problems, perhaps with specialized vocabulary, where everyone is uncomfortable about the three-way communication.

For a bilingual person to act competently as an interpreter requires enhanced 'bilingual skills', as well as training in 'interpreting skills', plus consideration of the 'interpreting role'.

Setting up situations without cognizance of these matters will inevitably lead to difficulties and probably to fallacious assumptions about, for example, the 'usefulness of interpreters for speech therapists'. Suggestions on how to avoid setting up such situations is discussed later in this chapter and will alleviate some of these difficulties. However, adequate training of both the 'interpreters' and their 'users' (e.g. speech therapists) would give bilingual clients a professional service.

Bilingual service provision within speech therapy in the UK is rare. Currently speech therapists spend much time and energy in locating available bilingual volunteers to assist. This is frequently unsuccessful. The lack of agency knowledge and training usually means it is unsatisfactory too (Abudarham, 1984). This situation is similar throughout the UK (Barnett and Stokes, 1985). Speech therapists in the USA in some states train bilingual staff as bilingual para-professionals, but again this is an *ad hoc* and problematic solution (Mattes and Omark, 1984). Speech therapists in India are still seeking solutions (Moffatt, 1985), as indeed they are in Sweden.

Having discussed models of bilingual service provision, and the need for training in interpreting skills, let us now move on to examine the specific tasks involved in interpreting.

SO WHAT IS AN INTERPRETER?

The *Oxford English Dictionary* defines an **interpreter** as 'one whose office it is to translate the words of persons speaking different languages, especially orally, in their presence', and that to translate is 'to express the sense of a word or sentence in or into another language'.

In this section we will look at the task of interpreters, giving consideration to skills required to perform the tasks involved, mentioning the styles and types of interpreting there are, and the training that is necessary. This concludes with a brief discussion of the role of interpreters.

The interpreter's duty is to the communication process, having the responsibility to ensure that two people are communicating with each other. Thus the task is to transfer the message uttered by one speaker to the recipient, and then to transfer the subsequent message of response. In order to do this, the interpreter has, first, to have understood the message; secondly, she has to be able to translate it accurately into the appropriate language, where accurate translation does not mean literal translation; and finally, to transfer the message to the listener, while monitoring that the listener is receiving the message.

In order to carry out this task, the interpreter will need to have good **interpersonal and communication skills**. It will also be necessary to have particularly good bilingual skills, together with biliteracy and biculturalism. Perhaps less immediately obvious and frequently overlooked is the need for the interpreter to have a well-developed auditory memory with excellent powers of concentration and attention. Conference interpreters have a break every 20 minutes, because of these demands on concentration.

There are three different **styles of interpreting** that may be adopted according to the needs of the situation: word-by-word, sentence-by-sentence or paragraph-by-paragraph conveying summaries or the gist of the messages.

Similarly, there are three different **types of interpreting**: consecutive, simultaneous and double.

Consecutive interpreting, as the term implies, means that the interpreting occurs in a sequence such that the speaker speaks, the interpreter transfers the message, the listener responds, the interpreter transfers the message, and so on. **Simultaneous interpreting**, meanwhile, is where the interpretation is occurring while the speaker continues speaking. The advantage in this is that the communication flow between speaker and listener is not interrupted. This is the style of interpreting often used at conferences where headphone sets are looped into a system with a particular interpreter and language. It is also a useful method for the interpreter to use in a situation of emotional outburst, where a distressed client is pouring out troubles, as there is no need to pause for the interpretation to catch up, thus the flow of feelings is not interrupted. Simultaneous interpreting can be whispered to the listener, so as not to distract the speaker. Simultaneous interpreting is obviously demanding work in a dialogue, so there can also be **double interpreting** (i.e. two interpreters), one for each 'side' of a dialogue. Whispered simultaneous double interpreting may well be a useful means in, say, a psychiatric social-work case requiring marital counselling. Double interpreting is useful in lessening the intensity of the workload on a sole interpreter, which will reduce errors and maintain a high standard of interpreting for a longer time period. It can be particularly helpful in international political discussions. However, consecutive interpreting can also be useful in such situations as it gives each side greater time to reflect before speaking.

Clearly, the task and skills required in interpreting are complex. They are also generally underrated. **Training** is essential. The few community interpreter training courses that exist (Institute of Linguists, London Interpreting Project) tend to take up to a year, and produce a truly high (and as yet little witnessed, or seen by speech therapists) degree of professional competence. The content of a training course needs to contain information on the agency (police, social work, housing, education welfare, etc.) and its specialist subject area for whom the student interpreters would be training. The training course must allow for practising the skills involved in interpreting such as memory, selecting correct vocabulary and phraseology for frequent phrases, etc. The student interpreters must be trained to interrupt and ask for clarification or elaboration if they do not understand part of a message, for if they do not understand it, they cannot translate or transfer the message. The training must also involve training for those who will be collaborating with the interpreters.

The **role** of the interpreter in the community setting needs to be clarified, as explained earlier. However, interpreters are beginning to get their work established as a profession in its own right. The (trained) interpreter's role should be regarded therefore as a co-professional rather than an assistant. The prime responsibility of the interpreter is to ensure that two people are communicating with each other, thus the interpreter remains impartial with loyalty to neither 'side', but to the communication process itself. It is also part of the interpreter's role to suggest to either party, when appropriate, where there may be a cultural difference causing misunderstanding or irrelevant questions (e.g. 'Perhaps it would be more useful to you to ask about the role of the grandmother?'). Quite how far the interpreter is to be a 'cultural attaché' is determined by their professional judgement as to whether such intervention is necessary for the communication process. Finally, confidentiality is an essential part of the role.

We have seen that there is a need for bilingual service provision in speech therapy, but that resources are scarce. We have also seen that the skills involved in interpreting are complex and require training to be developed properly. We will go on to consider how we can use the knowledge of these points to make optimum use of our current resources. Careful time management, planning and preparation are keys to success in this.

WORKING WITH 'INTERPRETERS' IN SPEECH THERAPY

WORKING WITH 'INTERPRETERS' IN SPEECH THERAPY

In this section we are concerned with how speech therapists can assist lay bilingual people to collaborate in speech therapy sessions to the best advantage for all parties involved. We will consider issues in location, selection, rejection and preparation of 'interpreters', then discuss how to conduct a speech therapy session with an interpreter, and, finally, consider the matter of payment.

Good contact places for locating bilingual people who may be willing to assist one are the local community groups (e.g. The Pakistani Women's Welfare Association, The Turkish Cultural Association, The Chinese Community Centre, etc.). They may know of people willing to assist, or they may employ someone specifically for this purpose. Community groups vary in size, security of funding, resources, organizational structure, duration of existence and political philosophy. Also many boroughs, and some education authorities (notably the ILEA) have established local interpretation and translation agencies. These, again, vary in their sources of funding and the width of their brief. Consequently, some will be able to provide interpreting facilities for anyone who approaches them with a need within a given set of languages, whereas others may be limited to working with local authority agencies and thus not for health authority agencies. Most such interpreting and translation agencies have no training, have variable selection criteria and little clarification of their employee's role.
Where one has options as to who to ask to assist as interpreter the following **selection criteria** should be considered:

1. (a) Ensure that the interpreter and client speak the same **language**. This may seem an obvious point, but it is surprisingly frequently overlooked — e.g. 'Oh, Mr X is from Cyprus, he'll interpret for us', quite missing that Mr X speaks Greek and the client speaks Turkish; similar comments are made about the 'Indian languages'. It is also helpful if the same **dialect** of the language is spoken, as there can be unhelpful prejudices with regard to dialects of differing status, which may well impede or distort the communication. Certain **language combin-**

101

ations are more likely to be present than others in one speaker, for reasons of geography and/or religion — e.g. Turkish (L1) and Greek for Turkish Cypriots, but not necessarily Greek (L1) and Turkish for Greek Cypriots, and similarly Urdu and Punjabi, Urdu and Bengali, but not Bengali and Panjabi. Obviously there will always be exceptions to such generalizations.

(b) Where the 'interpreter' has two or more languages, are they spoken well enough to ensure satisfactory 'interpreting'? Perhaps one language is only used in a very restricted way — e.g. religion, reading, unusual dialects? Thus they may be fluent in one and just able to 'get by' in the other. This may present particular difficulties in certain situations — e.g. most languages have colloquial terms for certain illnesses or parts of the body with which the 'interpreter' may not be familiar. The 'interpreter's' **linguistic abilities** are clearly of importance in both languages. This is relatively easy to establish for their English, but less so for their other languages. One is likely to need assistance with this.

2. In some situations the gender, religion, class and age should influence the choice of 'interpreter'.

(a) Many Asian clients may find it difficult to speak freely about intimate matters with members of the opposite **gender**. This may be particularly significant in cases involving relationship difficulties — e.g. in voice work or more simply in discussing pregnancy and birth details.

(b) The 'interpreter' may need to be matched or to have a good knowledge of the client's **religion** in order to make sense of unfamiliar behaviour or images used in descriptions of experiences — e.g. Hinduism and Islam have different views of mysticism and the supernatural.

(c) There may be a social **class** communication gap, or other unhelpful prejudices *re* class, caste or status.

(d) At times **age** can assume significance — e.g. in cases of intergenerational conflict on, say, child-rearing practices. Sometimes an interpreter is needed who can establish credibility with both parties.

3. Good **interpersonal skills**, particularly listening skills, are

essential for an interpreter anyway, but particularly so when working with impaired, poor or reluctant communicators.

4. At times people living in the same street or neighbourhood may have difficulty in ensuring **confidentiality**. This issue may need to be judged carefully.

5. Finally, it is necessary to check the time **availability** of the person and that they do not have conflicting commitments or priorities.

Occasionally someone's services to interpret will have been offered, yet they do not appear to be suitable. In such circumstances, for the client's sake, this potential 'interpreter' must be rejected. Such situations are difficult; it is therefore sensible to have this possibility in mind prior to meeting any potential 'interpreter'. An initial meeting should be set up for the speech therapist and 'interpreter', without the client, some days in advance, without entering into any commitment or discussion about the particular client. This provides a let out, so that general aspects of speech therapy can be discussed during the early part of the meeting. This meeting can then be curtailed sooner if the person does not seem suitable with 'Thank you, we'll be in touch when necessary'.

This initial 'no-commitment-yet' meeting is an essential part of preparation for future collaboration. There are three major points to be discussed. Such a meeting is likely to take an hour, and the therapist will need to be well prepared as there will be much for the potential interpreter to absorb during this meeting, thus the more digestibly it is presented the better. First, speech therapy must be explained, its purpose, role, types of liaison, and so on. Secondly, there is a need to outline the variety of types of communication impairment, its multifarious causes and therefore the differing means of assessing the difficulty. Finally, the roles of the therapist and 'interpreter' need discussion and clarification, so that both are clear about their mode of collaboration and what to expect from one another. It is possible the therapist may feel threatened by the presence of a co-worker in the session, who is able to understand all that is being said. It is necessary for the therapist to be aware of her feelings on this. It is also necessary to ensure the 'interpreter' feels comfortable with the therapist and potential clients. If unrealistic demands are made of the 'interpreter' by both sides, she may feel 'squashed' between therapist and client. For example, the client may say 'Don't tell the therapist this, but ...', or the therapist may make irrelevant or value judgement asides, or either might suggest 'Of course, she will go to the housing department with the family tomorrow, and then to the DHSS on Friday to interpret there, too — won't she!' Strategies for assisting the 'interpreter' out of awkward situations like this need to be worked out. It is important to make it clear at the beginning of the session that everything said by either party will be interpreted, and that confidentiality is assured.

Conducting the session — it is necessary to discuss a session with the 'interpreter' beforehand for about 10 minutes. This is to discuss the type and style of interpreting to be used, the seating arrangements and the purpose of the session. If the 'interpreter' is expected to assist in assessment during the session, then this preliminary meeting will need to be much longer in order to enable discussion of the purpose, type and method of assessment that has been chosen and to give the 'interpreter' a chance to practise, obtain feedback and ask questions. There are four main aspects to consider during the session itself, namely establishing rapport, eye contact, seating arrangements and giving clear messages:

1. Establishing **rapport** is essential to good communication in any situation, but particularly so in situations involving 'interpreters' with poor communicators and heightened anxiety levels on all sides. It is the responsibility of the therapist to ensure that she has established good rapport with the 'interpreter' prior to the session, that she organizes seating and eye contact, so that she is then able to establish optimum rapport with the client given lack of direct verbal communication, but that also she encourages the 'interpreter' and client to establish good rapport with one another. The essentials of 'small talk' before the session proper begins must not be overlooked, within which must be the clarification of the respective roles of all concerned, and assurance of confidentiality.

2. **Eye-contact** is a crucial part of communication. When communicating via an 'interpreter' in a speech therapy session, it is probably better to maintain eye contact with the person with whom the therapist is speaking rather than with the 'interpreter'. It is also the therapist's sole means both of monitoring the reaction of the client and of observing the client's non-verbal communication. Clearly, the

therapist must discuss her intended use of eye-contact with the 'interpreter' prior to the session, so that it is understood and there is no offence.

3. There is no right or wrong way to arrange the **seating**. This will alter according to the relationships of those involved, the shape of the room, and so on. Sometimes it will be preferable to have the seating arranged in a circle with everyone equally involved; at other times it will be preferable to place the 'interpreter' slightly further away, out of the direct line of vision of therapist and client; and at still other times it may be preferable for the therapist to be removed from the situation — e.g. when the 'interpreter' is eliciting a language sample from a $3\frac{1}{2}$-year-old child. A useful tip is for the therapist to consider how she would normally have seated herself relative to the client and family if there were no 'interpreter'. This is because if the therapist is attempting to establish rapport with a client and family with whom she can only communicate non-verbally, it is essential that she does not place the 'interpreter' such that this will physically be lessened or impeded. For example, if the therapist would normally sit next to the $3\frac{1}{2}$-year-old to point things out or give reassuring touch or smile, then this proximity must be maintained.

4. While the session progresses, the therapist must at all times be aware of the complexity of the 'interpreter's' task and ensure that she is phrasing her messages clearly and unambiguously such that they are easy for the 'interpreter' to decode and then to re-encode in the other language. If at any time the 'interpreter' does not understand the therapist (or client), it is essential that she feels comfortable enough to say so and to ask for clarification of what the therapist (or client) is saying such that she is able to transfer accurately the intended message. This should be emphasized at each pre-session discussion. It is crucial, but it can be extremely difficult for the 'interpreter' to do.

There needs to be a short (5 minutes or so) **debriefing** meeting after the session to clarify any misunderstandings, check whether any aspects of your collaboration need modification and to discuss any administrative procedures such as timing of other sessions, translating appointment letters, payment, and so on.

The matter of **payment** for someone's time and skills must not be ignored. If employed by an interpreting agency, or if interpreting duties is part of the person's job description within a community organization, then they are presumably already being paid for this work — though this should be checked. However, this is rarely the case. The agency may wish to charge the speech therapy department for its services. Where the 'interpreter' is an individual not within such an agency, as is more usual, then payment directly via speech therapy budgets can be difficult; however the 'interpreter's' travel expenses can generally be claimed via the therapist's travel claim form, and arrangements via petty cash can be made for payment of fees.

Having discussed how speech therapists and lay bilingual people can most constructively collaborate given current resources and skills, let us now consider a model of bilingual service provision for speech therapy for the future — bilingual facilitators.

BILINGUAL FACILITATORS

In the long-term, speech therapy departments need to be looking towards a more satisfactory and less *ad hoc* solution to bilingual service provision such as the employment of bilingual therapists and **bilingual facilitators**. It is ironic that other services are already bridging the communication gap, yet speech therapy lags behind, despite its need being arguably greater. This is primarily due to the paucity of speech therapy funding, but is also partly due to the different levels of recognition within speech therapy of this need; and it is also due to the complexities involved in this, in that speech therapy requires more than interpreting and more than a bilingual aide.

Here we look at some of these complexities, the practical and ideological issues to be considered, and suggest one possible model, namely the bilingual facilitator, as one solution.

Making the case for bilingual post creation

The following points are pertinent whether one is considering employing bilingual therapists (although there are also additional issues involved in that, which belong in a separate discussion), bilingual facilitators as outlined here, or some other form of bilingual service provision. Statistics on the numbers of bilingual referrals as a percentage of the caseload, and across each language spoken in the district, need to be collected and collated. In some areas local authorities or education authorities have such statistics for the general population which are helpful in showing trends and comparisons. It is easier to make the case in a district where one language is particularly dominant, yet arguably the need for trained bilingual assistance will be even more necessary in linguistically diverse populations where therapists may have up to 40 different languages on their caseloads and thus cannot be expected to know much about any of them.

Similarly, the current provision that a speech therapy district is able to provide in terms of professional service should be monitored, including how much care and time is spent on seeking suitable *ad hoc* bilingual assistance and thence therapists' and clients' feelings of satisfaction or otherwise in management of such cases.

In making a case for new post creation one needs to be clear about the role to be established as this will, in part, determine the qualities considered necessary in deciding selection criteria and the content, method and duration of training. It must be stressed that in speech therapy we need much more than 'bilingual volunteers', that remuneration for invaluable skills is essential and that those trained and employed for this purpose should have future career routes opened, otherwise we will not attract the calibre of staff needed.

It may well be the case that within each district the number of bilingual referrals for any one particular language expressed as a percentage of the entire population appears small. It is all too easy and wrong to then dismiss 'the problem' as 'not being a priority here'. Across parts of some regions or districts it is unquestionably a priority. It is likely that languages and numbers in neighbouring districts will be similar and thus it would be possible to share bilingual service provision costs and staffing with other districts.

Full- or part-time or sessional employment?

Full-time employment is preferable, that is the creation of full-time posts, although these may be job-shared. It is preferable because the alternative would be to have a speech therapy department staffed mainly by white speech therapists who would probably be full-time staff, particularly in the more senior positions, while the bilingual facilitators (almost by definition) will be ethnic minority staff. So to create specific part-time posts which would inevitably, although incorrectly, be viewed as subsidiary and of lower status for ethnic minority staff, within a mainly white, middle-class professional department of mostly full-time posts, is unsound practice. It would not enhance good working relationships and would be contrary to advice given by bodies such as the Commission for Racial Equality. Part-time-only posts do not create opportunities for bilingual facilitators to advance careerwise. To expect the calibre of person needed to do this complex type of work to train for part-time, dead-end employment is shortsighted.

To overcome the difficulties posed by the smallness of numbers and scarcity of financial resources to employ full-time staff there are two possible, not necessarily mutually exclusive, solutions. First, staff could be employed at a supra-district level, thereby sharing the cost across two or three districts, as suggested above. Alternatively, staff could be employed at supra-professional level, that is to train and employ bilingual facilitators to work with speech therapists and, say, educational and/or clinical psychologists. With both notions there are practical issues that will need careful attention, such as timetabling, to whom the bilingual facilitators are ultimately accountable and who holds the purse-strings. There are advantages and disadvantages to both but, on balance, the second option is probably preferable. This is because it would automatically create a more varied job, plus the potential for the bilingual facilitators of wider career development choice. It would also assist the creation of independent status rather than having 'assistants' attached to one department, and it also means that less time would be spent in travelling across a wider geographical area and that more time could be spent actually doing the job. A separate aspect to the advantages of a joint project with psychologists is that of funding. This is because psychologists are employed by education or social services and are thus eligible to apply for Section II funding (*Local Government Act 1976*, forms available from the Home Office), which is not open to health authorities but which is a particularly good source of funding for such work. A further advantage to a joint scheme is that it may have a beneficial side-effect in causing psychologists and speech therapists to work more closely together, promoting a clearer understanding of one another's roles, concerns and modes of working.

The role of the bilingual facilitator

This will be dependent, in part, upon consideration of the above as to whether they are working for professions other than speech therapy. Within speech therapy the role of the bilingual facilitator will be threefold:

1. To assist in bridging the communication gap between the therapist and client — i.e. interpreting and advising on cultural aspects, plus translating letters, reports and advice leaflets;
2. Assisting in the diagnostic process by having sufficient understanding of testing rationale and procedures to administer items for assessment of comprehension levels and to be able to elicit language samples from reluctant, poorly communicating 3-year-olds and to note down the responses;
3. Assisting the therapeutic role in carrying out, say, a language programme under the direction of the speech therapist.

The speech therapist's role, in the above, is to put together the items gleaned from the case history in role 1 and the communication behaviours sampled in role 2, with her in-depth theoretical knowledge of speech pathology and related disciplines, to arrive at a diagnosis and a plan of remediation for role 3, from her training in therapeutics and linguistics. This plan in role 3 is then put into action by those appropriate according to the language(s) involved, with the speech therapist then monitoring the progress made and modifying the remediation strategies as required.

The role of the bilingual facilitator for other professions is best decided by those professions involved. It seems likely there will be certain core components that would be similar across professions. These could be stressed in the training.

The selection criteria for bilingual facilitators

This would remain similar to those outlined in the previous section, in that the potential bilingual facilitator must be bilingual, biliterate and bicultural, with good interpersonal skills. The Institute of Linguists has produced a Bilingual Skills Certificate (Institute of Linguists' Educational Trust, 1987), which is a useful means of establishing the level of a person's skills in two languages, both orally and written, being at about a functional A-level standard. Assistance will be needed from community group representatives in considerations of 'biculturalness'.

The training for bilingual facilitators

This needs to be considered carefully as to the following.

1. The content and breadth of the course;
2. the training methodology and number of students per course;
3. the involvement and training of the professionals who will be working with the bilingual facilitators;
4. the staffing, cost, funding and duration of the course.

(a) The **course content** will need to cover the development of interpreting skills, understanding of the basic principles and rationale of assessment procedures, some therapeutic principles, counselling techniques vs advice-giving, their role with its responsibilities and limitations and, finally, speech therapy (and psychology) liaison networks. It is the speech therapist's role to know about communication disorders and pathologies, and language development theories; however, some knowledge of this will be useful for the bilingual facilitator. The wider the training is, the more options for the future there are open to the students — e.g. as to whether they move into psychology or speech therapy as a profession, or move more into interpreting as a profession.

(b) A useful **training method** for developing the skills needed in interpreting, such as memory, concentration and selecting the correct vocabulary and phraseology to convey the message, is to have the students listening to a talk on, say, language comprehension and then requiring them to paraphrase, in the other language, what they have just heard, say, every three or four sentences. It is necessary to have more than one student per language, so that discussions as to the best way of interpreting certain phrases can arise, and so that gradually a bank of useful terms and their counterparts, known as a 'term bank', can be compiled for future reference. This method of training interpreting skills while giving information is very useful in (i) assisting rapid learning of course content theory, (ii) helping develop concentration and memory skills, (iii) promoting discussion of concepts and development of the term bank, and (iv) being an immediate interpreting practice.

(c) Role-play is another useful device in this training for three reasons. First, it is a means of training the speech therapists and psychologists simultaneously with the bilingual facilitators. The speech therapists/psychologists will learn to appreciate a little more the complexities involved in interpreting, thus subsequently working with realistic expectations. More important, they can learn to improve their skills of making their messages clear. Speakers who wish their utterances to be interpreted accurately must make their messages as clear as possible. Similarly, it will provide the students with practice in interrupting when they have not understood a concept or jargon-term and asking for clarification. Secondly, such role-play will provide good varied, realistic work-models for the trainee bilingual facilitators, who can practise altering their style of speech according to the gender or age of person being interpreted for, and then discuss this in the company of other students. Thirdly, it provides both speech therapists/psychologists and student bilingual facilitators with the opportunity to clarify their roles in working together.

(d) Such a **training course** will need a high staff–student ratio and more than one student per language. The duration of the course should probably be spread over two or three terms for less than 20 hours per week and with practical placements. A recognized certificate should be developed for award upon successful completion of the course. Adult education institutes and local colleges of further education are likely to be interested in assisting with the course, and Section II funding could be a means of financing it.

THE WAY FORWARD

We can improve our utilization of current resources by increasing our understanding of the complexity of skills involved and clarifying our expectations. However, we need to move towards more adequate bilingual service provision which will involve at least six stages:

1. Collating statistics and making the case;
2. Determining the role desired, supra-professional or supra-district;
3. Development and financing of training courses;
4. Development and financing of local posts;
5. Monitoring and evaluation of local schemes;
6. Research furtherance and application.

Current provision is lacking and current expectations of 'interpreters' is unrealistic. The lay bilingual people currently being asked to assist as interpreters are not trained in overt linguistic analysis of their own language, nor language acquisition of this language, nor in testing procedures and rationale, nor in therapy techniques — nor could they be. There is much more research yet to be done. The establishment of bilingual facilitators might be one way of beginning to address these matters. (For further reading, see Ahmed, 1982; Baker and Briggs, 1975; Campbell, 1986; Corsellis, 1984; Malik, 1987.)

8

Linguistic Assessment Procedures for Bilingual Children

Jane Stokes and Deirdre M. Duncan

INTRODUCTION

In Chapter 1 a parallel was drawn between the researcher's methodological constraints and the challenges facing the practitioner in assessment. The variety of subject variables, data collection, analysis frameworks and aspects of language to investigate are shared by both researcher and practitioner. This chapter will look at the issues facing the practitioner, particularly the speech therapist, when assessing the potentially bilingually language impaired child, and the informal and formal techniques she may use in assessment. Finally, modification of first language (L1) English tests and the devising of new bilingual tests will be discussed with specific reference to two example cases.

BILINGUALISM: A CHILD COMPONENT

Subject variables include gender, social class, learning ability, medical and family history, and mono/bilingualism, as well as the emotional and motivational set of the subject. All the aspects of the subject are important (and none more important than another) because they all contribute to defining the uniqueness of the child involved. With some language-handicapped children one or more of these aspects may be highlighted — e.g. slow learning, emotional trauma or hearing deficit. The practitioner would acknowledge this in her language assessment protocol and seek additional assessment for the child from the psychologist, paediatrician or audiometrician.

Bilingualism is set among the subject variables rather than apart from them since it plays an intrinsic part in the subject's language and overall development, just as much as do learning ability and emotional equilibrium and the rest. Bilingualism — having or acquiring an additional language — is not a superimposed aspect of the child (see Chapter 2). It does not mean that the children developing two languages are innately different, or that by developing two languages they will become different. Being bilingual may contribute to, and precipitate the development of, different perspectives, concepts and sensitivities. The advantages of being bilingual are well documented (Abudarham, 1987).

In the same way, developmental difficulties which arise in the emerging bilingual will not be due to innately based differences from monolingual children. That is, learning difficulties, or whatever difficulty, do not arise from being an emerging bilingual. The (learning) difficulties exist apart from being bilingual (Bruck, 1984, p. 127) as the following case study shows:

Manjeet, a six year old Sikh girl, presented with mildly delayed expressive Panjabi and moderately delayed expressive additional English. Her non-verbal work was above average. Shortly after starting intensive group therapy, a behaviour problem was identified. After three months of therapy her expressive Panjabi and English were within the normal range, whilst her behaviour problem persisted.

The aim of language assessment must be to identify linguistic abilities and disabilities and to offer diagnosis.

When it comes to assessing a developing bilingual child presenting with language handicap, the same thorough assessment protocol can be implemented as with a monolingual child. If other agencies are required, then the child should be referred. The principles of assessment can be followed and standard practices, such as observation, mother/parent–child interaction, taping and transcribing a data corpus, linguistic and phonological analyses can be carried out (see Chapter 9).

The most important point is that these procedures must be carried out in both (all) the child's languages. It is only by having a grammatical and communicative profile in both (all) the languages of the child that a statement about her linguistic abilities and disabilities can be made with any degree of certitude.

The ways of organizing linguistic assessment have been discussed in Chapter 2. The requirement of a bilingual co-worker, if the assessor is not bilingual in the child's languages, has been clearly put. Other commonly met problems reflect the lack of resources in this field of work. Information about developmental features of many languages is not readily available to us — e.g. Vietnamese, Tagalog and Gujerati — although more research is being done on developmental aspects of languages other than English — e.g. Spanish, Irish, Welsh, Panjabi and Bengali. There are few standardized tests for bilingual children in various aspects of language; some that are available are discussed later.

Assessment needs of the bilingual child

The assessment needs of the bilingual child are essentially the same as those of the monolingual child. Regardless of the language(s) spoken by the child, the aims of assessment of her communication abilities remain the same:

1. To investigate the child's communication abilities in one or more specified areas of language (phonology, syntax, semantics, pragmatics or non-verbal skills);
2. To obtain a profile of the child's language which can serve as a relative statement of normality, or as a baseline for comparison before and after therapy;
3. To assist in making a differential diagnosis between communication disorder and other disabilities;
4. To describe a child's functioning in terms of her strengths and weaknesses, in order to design appropriate treatment and management;
5. To identify a child's educational needs in relation to her communication abilities, so that necessary resources may be organized to support the child in school;
6. To distinguish between the child with a communication disorder (i.e. with difficulties handling language receptively and expressively), and the child from a minority language background who is experiencing problems in expressing or understanding English, or other majority language.

This can be illustrated by the following case study:

Rubel, a 3-year-old child of Bengali (Sylheti) speaking parents, was referred to speech therapy by the doctor because of limited ability to use language. As part of a routine developmental check, the doctor had ascertained from the mother that he was not 'making sentences'. He had been attending an English day nursery since age 18 months. The aim of the speech therapist's assessment in this case was to investigate whether the problems reported by Rubel's mother were evident in Bengali (Sylheti), in English or in both these languages.

When a bilingual child is referred to speech therapy, the therapist must be able to detect whether the child's difficulties in communication are due to a basic communication disorder or to a limited exposure to English or other second language. It may be that a basic communication disorder is causing the child problems in acquiring the first, and also possibly the second, language. This need to establish whether there is an underlying communication disorder is central to the assessment procedure of the bilingual child. In order to select the children who would benefit from speech therapy intervention, the speech therapist must address the following questions:

1. Is the child acquiring communication skills in L1 and/or in L2 consistent with normal behaviour in her peer group?
2. Can speech therapy assist in recognizing, stating and fulfilling the child's needs, and if so, how?

It is often logistical problems which obscure and actually distort the challenge facing the practitioner in assessing and diagnosing the linguistic abilities and disabilities of the bilingual child. These include the resource of a bilingual co-worker; standardized assessment in the different aspects of language in the relevant languages, and for the relevant age-groups; and developmental information about the relevant languages. They may actually discourage the practitioner from applying these principles and practical procedures which could go some way towards providing a linguistic profile of the bilingual child. These will now be discussed.

Case histories

Excellent guidelines and details of case-history taking for use by the practitioner with a bilingual child have been given elsewhere

(Miller, 1984; Abudarham, 1987) and the reader is referred to these.

SOME ISSUES WITH MONOLINGUAL ASSESSMENTS WITH BILINGUALS

When faced with the task of assessing a bilingual, or potentially bilingual child, the speech therapist often feels inadequate. In the absence of sufficient developmental data on the minority languages, and with relatively few test procedures available, the practising speech therapist feels unable to make an assessment of a child's communication abilities. She may reach for the familiar tests and play equipment, partly because they are familiar and partly out of desperation, and in the absence of any established test procedures. Consequently, inappropriate play materials and tests can be used in informal and formal assessment. For example, a test which has been standardized on monolingual English speaking children may be used in the assessment of a bilingual child from a totally different population to that on which the test was standardized. Informal assessment may be made using play materials which are unfamiliar, even offensive, to the child and her family.

Formal and informal assessment procedures which rely on such shaky theoretical ground are unlikely to meet the needs of the child or of the speech therapist. These procedures cannot claim to fulfil the aims of assessment outlined earlier in the chapter.

Hasan, a 4-year-old child of Turkish Cypriot parents was assessed on a standardized monolingual English comprehension test. The practitioner scored his language level as being at a level of 1 year 7 months. This was relayed to the parents as evidence of Hasan's severe language delay. No assessment was attempted of the child's first and most familiar language, Turkish, and important decisions on the child's educational provision were made on the basis of a speech therapy report which stated that the child was delayed in his language ability by over two years. No reference was made in the report to the fact that the child had only been assessed on English, his weaker language.

A test standardized in English can only be used to assess the child's L2 English. The results obtained will reflect only the child's ability in L2 English, and this will clearly be influenced by the duration and type of exposure to English. It cannot inform about the overall language skills of the child.

ISSUES IN ASSESSMENT OF BILINGUAL LANGUAGE ABILITY

The assessment of the child's abilities in languages other than English will need to be adapted according to what facilities are available and whether the therapist has access to standardized assessment in languages other than English. Abudarham (1980) argues that a child from a bilingual background should be allowed to respond to a vocabulary test in either language for expressive and receptive vocabulary skills. In this way, he argues, the practitioner can obtain an overall picture of a child's lexical abilities across both languages. It may well be that testing each language separately does not give a true picture of the real bilingualism of a child, and there needs to be some way of assessing both languages together, and the possible effects of each upon the other. As each child's language environment is likely to be individual to that child, it will be difficult to develop standardized tests. The samples on which such tests could be standardized will be heterogeneous, and this will be discussed later. Therefore, we must look for other ways of assessment, making use of naturalistic data collection, spontaneous speech samples, probe techniques and the observation of parent–child interaction, which will be discussed below in more detail.

The speech therapist cannot hope to have a comprehensive knowledge of all the languages that she is likely to encounter. While speech therapists may steadily develop assessment procedures for the main minority languages spoken in the UK, Europe and the USA, there will continue to be other minority languages used by a substantial number of people but only in certain localized areas — e.g. Italian in Bedford in the UK, and Navajo in parts of the USA. The practitioner will continue to be faced with the difficulty of assessing a child whose first language is unfamiliar to her, for whom there is no interpreter/co-worker and about which language she has no information.

A 5-year-old child is referred to speech therapy. He is showing behaviour problems, and becomes frustrated when he is not understood at home. His parents speak Tiv (a Nigerian language) at home. His father or mother frequently return to Nigeria for two or three months at a time. They came to Britain when the child was aged 3½ years. The child speaks a mixture of English and Tiv with his younger brother. His parents report that the child is not using Tiv at a level appropriate to his age, and that his speech is not clear. The speech therapist is not able to discern whether this means that he is producing sounds and tones wrongly, omitting syllables or showing a language delay. There is no possibility of obtaining a Tiv interpreter.

In this situation the practitioner, particularly the speech therapist, will make full use of her abilities of accurate, systematic observation. She will be able to obtain information on whether a child initiates interaction, whether she responds to dialogue initiated by others, whether she uses gesture, etc. (Mattes and Omark, 1984, provide details of Observational Communication Inventories). The cultural diversity of non-verbal communication, the differing interpretations that can be put on gesture, and cultural attitudes to play have been extensively investigated and documented (Lieven, 1984).

Pragmatic language issues

This is the area, above all others, which demonstrates potential communication difficulties. It is the area, too, where variations between different languages and cultures which are likely to occur are most difficult to measure. Clinical observation of pre-school British Asian children suggests that early pragmatic development — up to the age of 3 years — follows similar stages to those outlined in the language development literature. For example, the range of illocutionary acts, such as pointing and showing, with or without vocalization, and turn-taking routines (Bruner, 1975), are demonstrated, as are the intentional use of early words to label, request, protest, greet, gain attention, etc. (Dore, 1975). Functional categories can be observed such as the instrumental, regulatory, interactional and other uses of developing language (Halliday, 1973), and conversational strategies such as verbal turn-taking, and the use of contingent queries and other means of topic maintenance are evident (Gallagher and Prutting, 1983).

As communication becomes more socially complex, such cross-cultural similarities appear to decrease, and assumptions need to be questioned. For example, Asian children may not be expected to initiate conversation with adults, and the clinician needs to establish with the family, through observation and discussion, which pragmatic processes normally operate. The young bilingual child has to learn not only appropriate social registers used with different listeners, but which different languages to use with them. This is an important additional pragmatic skill to assess: a child who demonstrates confusion in this area may well have underlying difficulties requiring remediation.

INFORMAL ASSESSMENT TECHNIQUES

Sampling

In many situations, particularly where a bilingual speaker is available to assist in the interpretation, a spontaneous speech sample can be obtained in a naturalistic setting (Lund and Duchan, 1983). There are some differences in the means of obtaining a recording of a bilingual child's speech, and the means of obtaining a monolingual child's speech sample. Tester bias will be a factor (Labov, 1969) and should be seriously considered as a strong influence on a child's language ability, which may be compounded in cross-cultural assessment. Practitioners may notice a marked difference between the sample obtained from a bilingual child when a person from a different culture is present to that obtained when she is not present.

Probe techniques

If a certain linguistic behaviour is to be tested, then it may be necessary to elicit these same behaviours by a more structured test. If, for example, a speech therapist wishes to investigate the ability of a child to mark the negative, she may artificially construct a situation where this is likely to occur — e.g. through using puppets who engage in dialogue, contradicting each other (Leonard, Steckol and Panther, 1983, provide examples of semantic probe techniques).

In obtaining an expressive, spontaneous speech sample the speech therapist will need something to compare the child's utterances with. Age-related linguistic information now exists on Bengali (Sylheti) and Panjabi (see Chapters 4 and 5) and will provide a framework for analysing a child's utterances in those languages. Even without this framework, however, a certain amount of information can be obtained from listening to a recording of a child's speech together with a native speaker of the child's language, who can then answer specific questions on the type of language used by the child.

STANDARDIZED ASSESSMENTS FOR THE BILINGUAL CHILD

There will always be controversy about the role and usefulness of the standardized test in language assessment. There are the antagonists who would argue that requiring a child to perform in a linguistically contrived context and to respond 'as — fast — as — you — can' will only yield an artificial and often low performance. Such tests may not provide a profile of performance, simply a numerical score. Further, although many testing procedures may be developmentally based, some offer a linguistically arbitrary collection of items (e.g. The Porch Index of Communicative Ability for Children (PICAC), Porch, 1974; The Reynell Developmental Language Scales (RDLS), Reynell, 1986). Finally, these tests may be standardized on one population group — e.g. North American white, middle-class university campus children — and yet used on other population groups which are sociolinguistically quite different — e.g. working-class children from the urban areas of England. They would argue in favour of more naturalistic data collection, linguistic analysis and, if necessary, the use of developmental (age stage) language information.

The protagonists of standardized language assessments would argue that standardized tests serve the function of separating the normal population from the disordered population. The purpose of testing a child is to discover her strengths and weaknesses **relative to her peers**. A numerical score permits statistical analysis which rules out elements of chance in the result and places the child's performance in relation to the performance of her peers. A numerical score can reveal little about the language processing of the child, but some tests do offer in addition some language profile and processing information (e.g. in phonology the Edinburgh Articulation Test, EAT). Furthermore, language testing is efficient in the sense that, in a short time, important information about the comparative language functioning of the child can be established. In this respect, screening assessments are important.

Standardization populations

The population on which bilingual language assessments are standardized arouses controversy. The debate is linked to other controversial issues, the main one being the 'dominance theory', which has been discussed in Chapter 1. There are those who advocate that tests for bilingual children should be standardized on the monoglot population of each language because the target language (TL) of the bilingual child is the monolingual's performance.

The argument against this is that to describe (prescribe?) the bilingual's TL in terms of monolingualism is arbitrary and artificial. The aim should be to describe what the bilingual child does, in terms of the grammar and functions of the L1 and additional language(s), as well as language-mixing and code-switching behaviours, and to base our assessments and norms on those descriptions. In other words, to standardize the assessments on the bilingual population. Moreover, since the language behaviour of bilinguals will vary from population group to population group, then (different) norms must be obtained for each group — e.g. Tex–Mex, Canadian French, English Panjabi, East African Panjabi, Creole and Black English.

Another argument in the standardization polemic supporting monolingual norms is that language norms, like intelligence norms, must be drawn from the general population, so that the child can be compared with her wider peer group. The argument against this is that in the case of an emerging bilingual child in L2 English, whose performance in English is compared with monoglot English children of the same chronological age, the emerging bilingual child can only fail. She may fail for one, two or three years, before 'catching up' with her monolingual peers, at an educationally sensitive period of her life. She may never 'catch up', depending on how the monolingual assessment and norms are drawn up. Furthermore, it can be argued that language does not function like intelligence and must be assessed differently. Whereas cognitive performance can be assessed non-verbally, language performance cannot.

The 'good' practitioner must choose her assessment procedure not necessarily on the basis of the above arguments, but more important, on the basis of needs of the child she must assess. She will also have to function within her own constraints, of time, resources and her own knowledge. The crucial points which formal standardized language assessment for the bilingual child must meet are, first, that it offers similar assessment in both (all) languages of the child, and secondly, that it has been standardized on the appropriate bilingual population.

Before considering using a standardized test with a bilingual child, the nature of her bilingualism should be investigated. Bilingual children are a heterogeneous group. Languages can be acquired simultaneously or consecutively, and one language, not necessarily the first to be established, may be the one preferred by the child. The pattern of language use (who speaks which language to whom, and when), the attitudes within the family and the status of the language(s) will affect the child's experience. There is considerable variation in the degree of switching or mixing of languages.

A bilingual child's overall language ability cannot be assessed using a test standardized on one language only. The child's responses in any language other than English must be recorded and taken into account. In a test standardized on English only, there is no formal means of doing this.

We believe that tests standardized on one language should not be translated into any other language without linguistic and cultural modification and restandardization on the appropriate bilingual population. It is often difficult to find exact equivalents of the English instructions in other languages, and the sequence of language development may be dissimilar. There will be differences in word order and in syntactic structures. Age equivalents and standard scores derived from the standardization in one language are not valid in any other language, and practitioners are doing the children a grave disservice by using them.

A standardized test may be useful in the assessment of the English abilities of a bilingual child, in that it may provide some qualitative information on the child's English and some guidance as to the areas needing remediation in English. There may be some argANTLR

justification for using the scores obtained as a baseline for comparison over time. We would stress that this is only an expedient, and it is no substitute for the use of tests properly standardized in other languages, and on bilingual populations of the type from which the child comes.

The information obtained by administering a test standardized on English to a bilingual child cannot provide a complete assessment of the child's language development. It can provide a useful indication of the child's English language abilities, which should be considered in conjunction with their bilingualism in the overall assessment of their communication skills.

MODIFICATION OF EXISTING LANGUAGE TESTS

In 1984, in the West Midlands, a project was set up to devise Panjabi scales for a mother-tongue (L1) English receptive language test, the Sentence Comprehension Test (Wheldall, Mittler and Hobsbaum, 1979). The aims of the project were to modify, adapt and, if necessary, extend the English design of the test to achieve accurate assessment of the understanding of the Panjabi syntax structures in 3.0–5.6-year-old Panjabi bilinguals. This project was embarked upon because there was no developmental data on the comprehension of Panjabi, yet the need for an assessment tool was pressing. A modified standardized tool was thought to be an acceptable way forward.

The procedures for adapting it are described here by way of an example. The problems of translation and the importance of restandardization on bilingual and monolingual populations are well demonstrated. The project team consisted of one of the test authors, a Panjabi–English bilingual teacher, a teacher of L2 English, a speech therapist and a professional artist.

After piloting an initial translation of the test on Panjabi bilingual children of 3.0–5.6 years, several modifications were made. The original test pictures were re-drawn, multiculturalizing and balancing them for gender and authenticity, as well as drawing new pictures for modified question stimuli. The same pictures were used for both language scales.

Translation

Certain items of English syntax did not translate meaningfully into Panjabi, for example, the English passive structure emerges between 3 and 4 years. In Panjabi the passive structure seems to be used only as a highly literary device. Items like this were omitted on the Panjabi scale. Translation often altered the syntactic structure being tested, so that certain picture stimuli tested one syntactic feature in English and another in Panjabi. For example, the post-modifying phrase in English translated to a pre-modifying phrase in Panjabi:

'The man with black boots is digging.'
'The black-booted man is digging.'

This yielded developmental information as well.

Lexis

Panjabi lexical constraints meant that pictures had to be modified, which affected the English scale as well. For example, the Panjabi word for 'ship' is also used to mean 'airplane', which is a much more familiar meaning for Panjabi children in the UK. So items with 'ship'/'boat' in them were given different lexis and re-drawn. Gender effects of Panjabi vocabulary meant that some items had to be re-cast and re-drawn. There were case structures in Panjabi, which were initially included, namely the ablative and oblique cases. In piloting these structures were not successfully handled by the children. The reasons for this are unclear; it could be that developmentally they emerge later.

Visual material

One interesting detail coming from this project clearly showed that good visual stimuli, that is pictures which accurately reflected the auditory stimuli, affect language performance. For example, the success rate for monolingual English children on one section for an early-emerging English structure was less than 30%. When the pictures were re-drawn, the success rate rose to nearly 70%, which was more in line with language development expectations for this structure.

The assessment was standardized on two population groups (in the English West Midlands). The English monoglot population set norms for the mother-tongue English scale. The Panjabi–English bilinguals set the norms for L2 English on the English scale, and mother-tongue Panjabi on the Panjabi scale. To interpret the results of the bilingual children the following questions were put:

1. Was the test sensitive to the development of the understanding of Panjabi structures?
2. Was the test sensitive to the development of the understanding of L2 English structures?
3. Were there structures which were outside any development trend?
4. Was there any correspondence between the structures understood in Panjabi and those understood in English?
5. Was there any correspondence between development of understanding in monoglot English and L2 English?

The development of comprehension in Panjabi

This assessment reflected a developmental trend of understanding of Panjabi structures — i.e. SV, SOV, tense (aux) + (participle), S Neg V, adj SV. Some structures seemed to be established already at 3 years (SV, SOV with the present tense and, to a lesser extent, past and future tense forms). By 4 years all the structures, bar two, are understood successfully, and by 5 years only one structure (pre-modification) is not meeting with overall success.

The development of comprehension in L2 English

Again, the test was able to reflect a developmental trend in the comprehension of L2 English. At 3 years the comprehension of English structures is predictably low, with success rates mostly at 20–30%. By 4.6 years there has been a big improvement and the success rate is over 50%. There remain only two structures which the five 5.0 and 5.6 years subjects find difficult (i.e. the passive and plurality).

Structures outside the developmental trend

On the English scale the passive structure is presented in the test as the reversible passive (e.g. 'The boy is being pulled by the girl'), which emerges developmentally later than the irreversible passives (e.g. 'The apple was eaten by the boy'). Plurality may have posed problems because, in the test, it is presented as a plural noun and plural aux + participle. It has been argued that the more prevalent the signals of plurality in a sentence, the more easily the plurality is understood (Harris, 1984). There does not seem to be an obvious explanation for the performance on this structure by the L2 English subjects.

On the Panjabi scale there are two (possibly three) structures which are not established at 3 years, and develop over the next two years. Adj. SV was handled successfully by only 50% of the 3-year-olds, but by 3.6 years 75% were handling it correctly and by 4.0 years it had a success rate of 90%. The other two structures which develop more slowly are the negative structure and the pre-modifying phrase. At 3 years the former has a success rate of 20%, and the latter no success at all. By 5.0 and 5.6 years they are beginning to stabilize.

Correspondence of Panjabi and English structures

There seemed to be a positive correspondence between the structures in the two languages, in that the success rate in understanding L1 Panjabi structures matched the success rate on the first language (L1) English scales. This seems to suggest that there might be some universal base for the comprehension of early-emerging structures across languages. Given that there were some exceptions to the developmental trend, this suggestion could only be cautiously endorsed.

Correspondence between L1 and additional English

There was a similarity in the developmental trend of the English scale for both population groups. This seems to be in line with studies on expressive language performance among L2 English subjects. Development patterns of L2 English follow, broadly speaking, those of monoglot English speakers. It is interesting to note that within two and half years of schooling (nursery and infant), bilingual children are achieving similarly, except for certain structures, to monoglot English children.

Finally, this project showed that with informed and sensitive work a comprehension test for one language could achieve successful and meaningful results in another language. It has also provided developmental information about the other language where no information previously existed.

EXPRESSIVE BILINGUAL LANGUAGE ASSESSMENT

Screening assessment

For many practitioners the initial linguistic assessment procedure might be a screening one, either a checklist or a screening test, in order to confirm the need for referral to speech and language therapy. It is not unusual for a practitioner to find herself having to assess several children such as a waiting-list, a nursery, a class or a school, in a limited amount of time. A screening test is usually standardized because the important point is the diagnosis of 'different in a delayed/deviant way from the peer group'.

In devising assessments of expressive bilingual language skills the same issues are raised concerning standardization populations, and the need to draw up accurate, relevant and appropriate test items in both languages. A project which aimed to devise such an assessment is now described.

The Sandwell Screening Test (SST)

The Sandwell Screening Test (SST) aims to screen the expressive grammar of English and Panjabi in bilingual primary school-children in the UK, aged 6–9 years. It assumes verbal comprehension is within the normal range, or only mildly affected. The English scale is based on the premiss that the development of L2 English follows the developmental pattern of first language English. It contains items which emerge within the first 36 months of language acquisition, as well as some later-emerging items (e.g. subordination clauses) and certain modals. At the time of devising the test this degree of developmental information was not available in Panjabi. So an informed 'guess' had to be made by the Panjabi members of the test team regarding what items of Panjabi grammar had been acquired by 6–9-year-old Panjabi speaking children in the UK. The standardization results both confirmed and rejected the accuracy of this 'guess'. Many of the features were established in 6-year-old Panjabi speakers and the results reflected developments on certain other features, particularly postpositions. By 9 years all the test features seemed established in expressive Panjabi (Duncan and Gibbs, 1987).

Each child is individually tested by being shown picture stimuli with accompanying questions. Only the subject can see the pictures which encourages the child to reply expansively and discourages deictic responses (e.g. pointing and/or saying such things as 'this', 'that', 'here', 'there'). The items are elicited in a flexible obligatory context. The screening test items in both language scales are marked on a simple error analysis (x/√); there are key features in each response. A grammatical item is marked once only, although it may appear several times in the subject's data corpus. Thus the final numerical score represents a qualitative number of vulnerable grammatical items rather than a frequency count of grammatical 'errors'.

The screening procedure may be used by any personnel familiar with test administration protocol. It is most important that both language scales are administered to the bilingual subject because the test offers differential diagnostic information. If the child's score is within the normal range on the Panjabi scale, but significantly below the norm on the English scale, then this child does not have a language acquisition problem *per se* but rather a problem with acquiring L2 English. If the child is significantly below the mean (−2SD) in both languages, then she is presenting with a language acquisition handicap. This is an important diagnosis to make. The types of cases are different, and they will be discussed later.

The main point to remember about tests is that they have specific parameters and cut-off points; this holds even more so for screening tests. It is most important that no assessment tool is used beyond its range. The SST will not, of itself, give information about a grammatical profile, in the sense of highlighting the linguistic processes and strategies which the child is using. It does give a data corpus, if the child's responses are tape recorded in both languages, which could be further analysed along descriptive linguistic lines, and a much richer picture of the child's linguistic functioning could be obtained. Familiarity with English and Panjabi grammar structures is obviously an essential requirement for such a procedure.

Selection for therapy

Following as full an assessment procedure as is necessary, a diagnosis must be made and the management and therapy requirements of the child stated. The key diagnosis to be made with a bilingual child must state whether the language problem concerns only the additional language or whether it stems from a fundamental language impairment mechanism, affecting the development of both languages. This diagnosis will influence management and therapy of the problem if it is at syntactic, phonological or semantic levels, and/or whether the child has additional or slow learning abilities.

Quirk, in his report on the speech therapy services in England and Wales, has given guidelines for the management by speech therapists of bilingual children:

> The speech therapist's role should not in normal circumstances go beyond assisting with the assessment of language development. But ... mastering English may in a small minority of cases mask a disability of pathological origin. These cases are, of course, precisely the concern of the speech therapist. (Quirk, 1972, p. 67)

If the child presents with a language development problem in L2 English only, the speech therapist must further differentiate the quality of the problem by deciding whether the various aspects of L2 English have a pattern of normal development in English, or whether the pattern is distorted in an abnormal way. For example, in phonology, Panjabi speaking children may take more time developmentally to expressively differentiate the phonemes/sounds [p] and [f]. This seems to be a 'normal' process in the acquisition of L2 English by Panjabi speaking children. Another example in morphological development is the differentiation of gender, and it seems to be 'normal' for Panjabi speaking children to take a few years to establish gender differentiation in L2 English.

Examples of abnormal patterns would be the presence of a lateral 's' in the L2 English phonology, the absence of all verb inflections, restricted clausal development and exceptionally slow development in L2 English. Where there is abnormal development in L2 English, there should be involvement of speech therapy management. Such cases, with appropriate care, often resolve quickly.

CONCLUSION

In this chapter we have discussed the wide range of issues relevant to the linguistic assessment of bilingual children. The assessment of ability in more than one language, the use of L1 English tests and their norms are clearly important for disciplines other than speech therapy. The outlined procedures have parallels in the fields of education and child health. We feel it is important that the various disciplines involved in assessment of bilingual children continue to work together to improve the service available to them and to meet the psychological and educational needs of the potentially bilingual child.

9

Intervention with Bilingual Pre-School Children

Farat Ara and Calla Thompson

BACKGROUND

Speech therapy intervention with pre-school children is on the increase, partly due to clinicians' greater knowledge and understanding of early child development, particularly language. This has not only helped to identify language breakdown in early developmental stages, but also to describe the stages along which therapy can proceed. Other professionals, such as paediatricians, psychologists and health visitors, are also referring children for speech therapy much earlier due to their increasing awareness of the speech therapist's role with very young children. Obviously early intervention has the benefit of remediation at the optimum age for language acquisition. This holds true for children who are exposed to more than one language, but there are additional issues to consider for these children such as sociocultural differences and the complexity of the linguistic environment. The fact that the majority of clinicians are monolingual but may be treating bilingual children from different cultures is another complicating factor. This chapter introduces the concept of speech therapy intervention with pre-school children, and sociocultural, socioeconomic, linguistic and psychological factors which are likely to affect the linguistic development of ethnic minority children are touched upon. In addition, we shall discuss assessment and management issues, and describe a speech therapy clinic set up for a specific minority population.

For the purpose of this chapter the **pre-school child** is defined as one who has not started attending full-time nursery school. The

132

age range will therefore vary between birth and 3–5 years. The main reason for using this definition is that the whole issue of bilingualism changes once the child starts a full-time nursery placement and is then truly exposed to the language of the majority culture.

This chapter is mainly concerned with children from a British Asian background, although the general principles may apply to other bilingual children. These children form a large and increasing population throughout cities in Britain (DHSS, 1981), and speech therapists are finding themselves increasingly responsible for the assessment and management of young children whose mother tongue is Panjabi, Bengali, Gujerati or Urdu.

The term **bilingualism** requires a special explanation when discussing pre-school children because they have not been formally exposed to English as a language for education. However, they can be exposed to a variety of languages from their environment, the quality and quantity of which is not necessarily constant during the first five years.

When seen by speech therapists, the majority of pre-schoolers, although potentially sequential bilinguals, are primarily monolingual, in that they are mainly directly exposed to one language, their first language (L1), but additionally receive passive exposure to the L2 from their surroundings (e.g. from siblings, television, etc.). However, the L2 is not directly spoken to them, thus they can be termed 'passive bilinguals' (Miller, 1984). 'Bilingual' is also used as a shorthand term to describe children who could be exposed to more than two languages (this will be discussed later).

INTRODUCTION

Pre-school children have, by definition, not yet been exposed to our major educational institutions, and remain embedded in, and largely influenced by, their families. It is accepted that language intervention with any pre-school child must be carried out within the context of their family; when working with ethnic minority children who are living in extended family networks within a majority culture not their own, the influence of the family may be particularly strong.

Sociocultural considerations are therefore as important as issues of language for the clinician working with pre-school bilingual children and their families, and the two cannot be separated. An awareness of different cultural traditions, particularly those relevant to the development of communication — such as child-rearing practices and family relationships — are necessary on a practical level when choosing the best settings, activities, assessors, languages and co-workers for the assessment and management of these children. Such an awareness will also help create the basis of understanding and co-operation needed in any joint venture between families and professionals. There may be differing assumptions about concepts such as the 'developing child', and expectations about 'medical intervention', which the clinician needs to explore sensitively during assessment.

An awareness of different cultural practices should not outweigh socioeconomic issues, which are also highly pertinent to this population. Asian families are particularly likely to have low incomes, work anti-social hours and live in the poorest housing with the highest number of dependants per working adult (CRE, 1978). As the Home Affairs Select Committee (1981) points out, such social deprivation is not exclusive to ethnic minority groups, but they do experience it disproportionately, and in conjunction with racial discrimination. Therefore, when a clinician considers matters like play opportunities at home, for example, the possible social factors, such as lack of space and money, will be as important as issues related to types of play and toys traditionally used within that culture.

On an interpersonal level the disruption of social relationships resulting from immigration should also not be underestimated. The splitting of the extended family network which successfully rears its children can lead, in some cases, to extreme isolation and lack of support and advice, and put strains on interpersonal relationships and communication within families (Commission for Racial Equality, 1978). The complex social and psychological influences liable to impinge on children's language acquisition and use need considering when determining possible language difficulties and planning intervention. Up until the present time, pre-school services within the community which might compensate for the extended family in this country — particularly mother-tongue playgroups and other support groups — have been too few, and too poorly used to be of significant benefit. Fortunately, this pattern does seem to be changing (DHSS, 1984), which is of interest to the language clinician.

Pre-school Asian children in Britain will, of course, sooner or later be exposed to, and learn, English. Happily, the time has passed when clinicians automatically assumed from this that *sooner* was always preferable. Now the importance of developing and maintaining the child's mother tongue is recognized for children's cognitive and communicative development (Cummins, 1979). Speech therapists are becoming increasingly aware of the linguistic diversity existing in multicultural Britain, and acquainting themselves with, for example, the social and semantic differences which are important when assessing language competence (Miller, 1984).

However, this does not mean that these pre-school children are simply either monolingual or bilingual. Although many pre-schoolers in Britain can, and do, exist without coming into direct contact with English (Wilding, 1981), they may nevertheless be exposed to a complex linguistic environment. In-depth investigation of this environment — i.e. the number, relative status and pattern of use of different languages, plus speakers' attitudes towards them — must be a priority during assessment and remediation.

In the end, the success of intervention with pre-school bilingual children will depend on each clinician's grasp of the cultural, socio-economic, psychological and linguistic issues involved, together with a willingness on her part to question her own values and assumptions. Generalizations are all too easy to make when working across cultural boundaries, and ethnic minority groups are by no means homogeneous in terms of economic, class or cultural background. Even within different groups, those originating from Bangladesh, Pakistan or India will show considerable variations. While remaining aware of general patterns, each child and her family needs to be considered individually.

ISSUES OF ASSESSMENT AND MANAGEMENT

When assessing any pre-school child's communication, criterion-referenced assessments, both pre-verbal and linguistic, which are based on a representative sample of the child's natural behaviour, are generally found to be the most useful (Miller, 1981). These can be supplemented by the few standardized assessments available (Reynell DLS, British Picture Vocabulary Scale, etc.), and used in conjunction with developmental checklists.

The gathering of a sample of natural communicative behaviour can be a delicate operation with this age-group; communicative competence is not a unitary and relatively constant ability centred on the child, but varies considerably according to the context and people involved (Mahoney and Seeley, 1976; McConkey, 1984). The most representative samples are therefore obtained in a variety of natural settings (home, playgroup) and with at least two different 'communicative partners' (family members, peers) (Prutting, 1982). Functionally, of course, there may be difficulties with the choice of setting for assessment, and an informal play-room in the clinic or nursery can be the most practical compromise. Free-play in the presence of a familiar person is the preferred medium of assessment, as it is a natural activity for the young child, and tends to increase verbal communication (Bloom and Lahey, 1978), as well as providing important additional information about the child's level of cognitive maturity (Lowe, 1975; McCune-Nicholich, 1981), non-verbal communication, comprehension and parents' preferred interactive style (McConkey, 1984).

Following from this, general management of language-delayed pre-schoolers will include encouragement of the child's own acquisition strategies, both cognitive prerequisites for language, such as auditory attention and selective listening, symbolic functioning, etc., and social prerequisites, such as joint focus, turn-taking, gaze behaviour for feedback, etc. The increased use of facilitation strategies normally used by adults with young children, for example, reduction of the length and complexity of their language input and frequent repetition and paraphrasing, will, if necessary, be encouraged in the adults surrounding the child (McLean and Synder-McLean, 1984; Bruner, 1975). The establishment or fostering of pre-verbal and verbal communication routines based on a shared focus and at a level appropriate to the child's functioning forms the basis for the development of language through generally observed stages (Bates, 1976; Bloom and Lahey, 1978). Intervention is carried out in truly interactive social situations, often at home with the child's family, or in groups of the child's peers, to ensure a broad range of natural communication.

ASSESSMENT AND MANAGEMENT OF THE BILINGUAL PRE-SCHOOL CHILD

Generally the same principles and rationale for assessment and treatment apply to culturally different children as well as to mono-linguals (Prutting, 1982; Miller, 1984). Naturalistic play-based observation of bilingual pre-schoolers with members of their families in a variety of settings gives a good picture, when backed up with a detailed case history and a social-communication questionnaire. However, with this group some methods need modifying, while others need special emphasis, particularly in the light of sociocultural differences and the complex linguistic issues involved.

1. **Criterion-referenced and standardized assessment**. As has been discussed elsewhere, knowledge of normal development in ethnic minority groups, especially linguistic development, is so sparse that establishing accurate criteria has not been possible. The clinician therefore has to rely on her knowledge of developmental patterns that seem to be *universal*, both pre-verbal and linguistic (Brown, 1973; Omark and Erikson, 1983). This is especially possible with young children at the stage of emerging language where there are considerable surface similarities — e.g. the progression from early vocalization to proto-words, one-word utterances and the linking of two words, etc. (Bloom, 1970; Slobin, 1970). The same universal principles have to be applied when planning treat-ment of language-delayed bilingual children. However, it is important for the clinician to bear in mind cultural differences in communication which may *not* be universal. Eye-contact between parent and child, and the initiation of conversation by the child with an adult, for example, may be discouraged in young Asian children past a certain age. Whenever the potentially subjective matter of making 'universal' assumptions arises with any child, the clinician must be scrupulously aware of such sociocultural vari-ables, and of her own attitudes towards them.

2. **Clinician's involvement**. Most clinicians are only too aware of the effect of the presence of a stranger on a young child's spontaneity. It has been pointed out, with some truth, that 2-year-old children have the pragmatic choice of speaking or clamming up in these situations, and often choose the latter. Therefore, it is par-ticularly important with young children that the effects of observer

interference are minimized during assessment. Ideally the least intrusive arrangement would be observation of the child inter-acting with family members, via a one-way mirror, remote-controlled video (CCTV) or unobtrusive 'fly on the wall' observation in the same room, together with the presence of a bilingual clinician. Of course, most clinicians currently have to rely on interpreters/facilitators, and the benefits and difficulties of this are discussed elsewhere (Chapter 7).

The exchange of information during assessment and manage-ment is usually two-way. When a clinician is dealing with a culture that is not her own, she may have to rely more heavily than usual on ideas and advice from the family, the bilingual co-worker and other members of the ethnic communities. This may range from specific information about what experience the child has had of various assessment objects, and what names are used for them, to general advice about social customs and taboos necessary for planning treatment.

Clear explanations of the purpose and procedures of speech therapy may also need to be made a particular focus, when shared cultural assumptions do not exist. For example, the process of therapy may need to be differentiated from medical treatment; and the rationale behind play-based therapy well discussed with families who do not have an existing concept of fostering children's development through definite stages. This is not to say, however, that a culturally imperialistic attitude is advocated, where unfamiliar practices are forced on families in a 'take it or leave it' way. But the reverse fear of such practices not being accepted by families can mean that clinicians sometimes fail to intervene when they could usefully do so (see discussion on 'play', below). Clinical experience shows that language intervention techniques can be successfully adapted for use with bilingual children. The adaptation needs to come from both sides; the clinician tailors her approach by considering the family's needs and they, in turn, may try out some of the unfamiliar suggestions she makes, as long as they understand the reason behind them, or see how they work during modelled therapy.

3. **Family involvement**. It is now common practice for young children to be assessed and treated within the context of their families. In particular, the importance of the mother–child relationship to the child's development (Snow, 1978) has made that relationship a focus for clinicians when assessing and fostering

young children's communication. The same focus applies to children from different cultures up to a point, but there is also a wide variation in child-care practices, and Asian children especially may have a number of main adult care-givers (grandparents, aunts, older siblings) once past infancy. The implications for this are several: the clinician needs to enquire about the structure of the often extended family network, to discover the patterns of decision-making and involvement with the child; she may need to obtain case-history information from other people besides the mother; and may need to involve other family members more in assessment and treatment. For example, watching children play with older siblings as well as parents, and actively involving them in language therapy, may be useful — as they may be able to play with the child more readily and naturally than the older members of the family. It has been observed that in Bengali and Pakistani families communication between siblings is often more natural and varied than parent–child interactions, which are more formal and less frequent. Often there is also the expectation that children should remain quiet in the presence of adults, which may confound the clinician's attempts to increase communication, unless she adopts a flexible view of whom to involve in treatment.

As different family members may speak different languages to the child, it is especially important to observe their separate and collective interactions with the child, to obtain a comprehensive picture of the child's social and language functioning. This information, of who speaks what language to whom under what circumstances, is vital for the language clinician. For example, the child's grandparents may speak Panjabi and the parents both Panjabi and Urdu — which is the medium for education in Pakistan. Therefore, the parents may decide to teach their children the higher-status Urdu, as well as communicating in Panjabi. If the child's older siblings attend school, English may soon become their dominant language, and the child may therefore be exposed to three languages. Under such circumstances, which are fairly common in British Asian families, the clinician cannot expect to advise that the child be exposed to just one language, without changing the family's natural pattern of communication.

Because more than one person is likely to be involved in therapy, it is often a good idea for the clinician to form a good relationship with, and gain the co-operation of, the most influential member of the family (usually grandparents or mother's in-laws).

139

This observation of protocol may help motivate the whole family to participate in therapy and, on occasion, overcome practical difficulties such as the younger female members not being allowed to attend clinic. To avoid diffusion of responsibility, when several people are involved in therapy, it may be appropriate for the most influential member of the family to supervise.

4. **Settings**. The relative merits of working at home or in clinic settings with pre-school children have been discussed elsewhere (Howlin, 1984; Spradlin and Siegel, 1982). Clinical settings may make observation and modelling easier as special recording and other equipment is to hand, but these, too, are unfamiliar, may be associated with medical treatment and may discourage participation. The home environment provides a more relaxed and natural context where intervention can involve all the family, and the use of everyday materials and the child's familiar toys. There may be drawbacks, such as noise and other disruptions, and home-visiting is time-consuming for the clinician.

Some additional practical considerations about settings may arise with bilingual children, again mainly related to working across cultural boundaries. The speech therapy clinic may be made as accessible as possible, with the inclusion of culturally familiar mother-tongue speakers and suitable materials, but it is still true that a mixture of social constraints, such as the limited movement of some Muslim women outside the home and limited knowledge of English language and customs, can make regular attendance difficult. The take-up of speech therapy provision has to be seen within the context of general access to other health and social facilities. Visiting the family at home is necessary for completing the picture of social relationships, languages spoken, etc., as well as involving the whole family in therapy, and can overcome attendance problems. It has been pointed out that confusion and suspicion can arise from the unfamiliar experience of professionals 'intruding' into home life, but in practice when the purpose of such visits is well explained, and the suitability of visitors (in terms of gender, class and language background, etc.) ascertained, then working in the home can be as successful with this as with any other group.

When dealing with monolingual language-delayed children, one management suggestion often considered, especially for the isolated child, is attendance at a general playgroup. In the UK this option may not be as freely available for the ethnic minority child as provision of mother-tongue playgroups is still inadequate for the population (DHSS, 1984). The language clinician considering therapy with groups of bilingual children is faced with similar constraints about settings. Imaginative compromises need to be, and currently are being sought, to make attendance at such groups more likely, for example, speech therapy input into existing mother–toddler groups, either attached to English as a foreign language (EFL) classes attended by ethnic minority women, or those set up by health visitors and link workers in the community, or those run in cultural community centres.

5. **Play**. Play-based assessment and intervention with monolingual children is fairly straightforward as the therapist can supply play materials based on her own cultural knowledge with some confidence as to their suitability. However, both the concept and methods of play may differ across cultures. For example, it may not be normal practice for parents and children to engage in mutual symbolic play, and there may be an emphasis on 'educational' rather than 'recreational' toys. Obviously clinicians do have to be aware of what the range of culturally normal play is, and to be especially sensitive to religious taboos such as orthodox Islam's prohibition against dolls and other representational materials. Clinical experience, however, suggests that many Asian children in the UK do have similar play materials to their monocultural peers, while others are willing to play with representational toys, even though these may be unfamiliar. As with all other issues, the clinician needs to remain aware of cultural possibilities, while always enquiring into individual practices within families. Traditions within ethnic minority cultures are not static, and rigid assumptions cannot be made, one way or the other. Little research data exists on the play experiences of British Asian children. One comparative study of interest (Child, 1982) of English and Asian pre-schoolers in playgroups found that there are some differences: the Asian children spent more time in the process of play rather than in the products; they preferred manipulative/constructive play (such as Lego, sand, etc.) to imaginative 'make-believe' play; required more adult direction; and initiated far less verbally to the adults present, not using them as a resource as did their white English middle-class peers. These patterns of play were obviously partly the function of social class differences as well as ethnicity, the last two points being also common to white working-class children.

Understandably clinicians may be wary about the value of introducing a possible alien concept, such as the assessment and treatment of communication delays through the medium of play, to
different cultural groups. However, as has been discussed above,
some monocultural intervention methods can be both useful and
successful, when adapted sensitively. The encouragement of play
may be particularly beneficial for Asian children living in the often
more isolated and less stimulating British social environment,
having come from more stimulating extended social networks.
When the compensatory benefits of play are discussed in this way,
families are often willing and able to try out unfamiliar activities.
The clinician does not have to rely on the usual symbolic doll play:
the process of play and intervention is more important than the
content, and a range of shared playful activities, such as hide-and-
seek and 'build and bash' games, shared constructional activities,
and football and other physical games may be appreciated (play
materials are discussed in more detail below).

6. **Linguistic issues**. The term 'bilingual' may be too simple a
description for this pre-school age-group, who have not yet been
exposed to the majority language at school, and yet may have had
varying degrees of exposure to it and other languages at home. The
presence of three or even four languages in the home is possible,
especially when members of extended families live in close
proximity. While bearing in mind that each child will be different,
there may be general patterns of language choice evident. Children
may be monolingual; 'passively' bilingual, where a second
language is heard indirectly but not spoken (e.g. Panjabi and
Urdu; Turkish and Farsi; Gujerati and Hindi); 'simultaneously'
bilingual, but where the quality and quantity of the different
languages are rarely equal; or 'sequentially' bilingual, when, for
example, the family moves country, or caregivers change, exposing
the child to other languages. Variables such as the age of the child
when this happens, the consistency of exposure and the psychological implications of such changes for the child and her family
are likely to have a strong bearing on the rate and quality of
language acquisition.

A model such as the one given above implies that languages
develop more discretely than is evident in reality. In practice, other
processes may also operate, such as lexical borrowing and code-
mixing. Some examples between Panjabi and English are:

Lexical borrowing: [ɹied bal kɪʈʰɛ vɛ]? = 'where's the red ball?', where 'red' and 'ball' are borrowed from English, rather than the purely Panjabi version [lal gɛnɖ kɪʈʰɛ vɛ]?
Code-switching: for 'Mummy, I don't want chappati, I want chips: [ʌmã mɛ̃ ɹɔʈɪ neɪ kʰanɪ. aɪ wɒnt sum tʃɪps]
Code-mixing: [mɛ̃ ɹɔʈɪ not it] = 'I don't want to eat chappati'.

These processes may be employed by speakers in the child's environment, the first two being particularly common. During assessment they will have to be identified in the environment, and differentiated from disordered language processes in the child. Borrowing and code-switching occur naturally in many young children's language. During management, code-mixing may need to be discouraged, if the child is showing difficulty differentiating language codes.

The phenomenon of the bilingual 'silent period' (Kessler, 1984) may differ, in the pre-school years, from the silence which sometimes occurs following sudden changes in environment or language input. British Asian families may make extended visits to the Indian subcontinent, particularly during their children's early years, to prevent disruption of schooling later on. Therefore, the young child may suddenly find herself exposed to a different language, or possibly a 'purer' version of her mother tongue from relatives, and will then have to readjust when returning to Britain. Alternatively, this can happen to a young child immigrating for the first time to Britain, when there is a sudden and sometimes total language switch within the family. The emotional effects of 'culture shock' on both child and family, combined with changes in language, can lead to a disruption in already-developing language, especially if the child is at the vulnerable stage of early language acquisition. The child's mother tongue is sometimes in danger of being lost, and advice about language input is particularly necessary.

The choice of language(s) used during intervention must ultimately remain with the child's family; as many pre-school children are 'passive bilinguals', the choice of their mother tongue is often a simple one. Families may need reassurance that they do not have to alter the natural balance of communication at home by teaching their child the majority language before entering school. However, the principle of 'consistently associating one person with one language' (McLaughlin, 1978) will need discussing if there is evidence that the child is being confused by extensive code-switching at home. In these cases, where the child is directly exposed to two or more languages, the same ideas concerning optimum language input can be implemented by different family members using different languages. This consistency of approach often seems more beneficial and more practical to achieve than attempts to reduce the number of languages in the home. Young language-delayed children can find it easier to process simple structures in two languages than lengthy, abstract utterances in one language.

Evaluation of different aspects of the young bilingual child's language is necessary in order to identify problems requiring intervention. As has been stated, enough universal similarities exist between different languages, particularly at the early stages, to make adaptation of principles pertaining to one group possible with other groups. Clinically we can assume, for example, that syntax, semantics and phonology develop along similar lines to those described for English speakers, (Brown, 1973; Munro, 1985) with obvious lexical and phonemic variations. This means that language profiles, giving an indication of the child's functioning in relation to developmental stages, can be constructed. Pragmatic language issues need special mention, for two reasons. First, this is the area above all others which demonstrates potential communication difficulties; and secondly, it is the area where variations between different languages and cultures which are likely to occur are most difficult to measure. Clinical observation of pre-school British Asian children suggests that early pragmatic development — up to the age of 3 years — follows similar stages to those outlined in the language development literature (Bruner, 1975; Halliday, 1975; McTear, 1985).

As communication becomes more socially complex, such cross-cultural similarities appear to decrease, and assumptions need to be questioned. For example, Asian children may not be expected to initiate conversation with adults, and the clinician needs to establish with the family, through observation and discussion, which pragmatic processes normally operate. The young bilingual child has to learn not only appropriate social registers used with different listeners, but which different languages to use with them. This is an important additional pragmatic skill to assess: a child who demonstrates confusion in this area may well have underlying difficulties requiring remediation.

A SPEECH THERAPY CLINIC FOR PRE-SCHOOL BILINGUAL CHILDREN

This clinic is housed in Manchester Polytechnic's Speech Pathology Department, and derives its clinical caseload from the Central Manchester Health Authority community. Although not exclusively a pre-school clinic, most referrals are in fact in this age-group.

There is a significant Pakistani, Indian and Bangladeshi population in Manchester: 3.35% of the total population have household heads born in these three countries. Of these, 1.74% have household heads born in Pakistan; nearly one-third of this population is in the pre-school age-group (OPCS, 1985). Although the figures quoted are for the whole City of Manchester, there is a higher density of Panjabi/Urdu speaking Pakistani, and Panjabi speaking Indian people within central Manchester (no figures available). Referral of pre-school children from this population to speech therapy is high (approximately 25% of total referrals). A special clinic for Panjabi/Urdu speaking children was therefore considered necessary.

Two speech therapists are involved in the clinic, one being a Panjabi/Urdu speaker already employed in the district and the other a monolingual English speaker. It was felt that the complex and relatively unexplored linguistic and sociocultural issues of bilingualism necessitated a joint approach. A large playroom and a smaller treatment room are available, connected by a remote-controlled video recording system; the provision of transport facilitates attendance, and the employment of a female driver especially overcomes social restrictions faced by some Muslim women.

Initially Panjabi or Urdu appointment letters, together with an English version, are sent to the family. Both parents are invited to attend for initial interview, and attendance of as many family members as possible is subsequently encouraged. It is common for siblings and grandparents to attend. This is particularly useful since the grandparents are often not only the most influential members of the extended family, but may also be the child's primary care-takers. The appropriateness of play-based assessment and therapy for pre-school children, and the necessity of utilizing culturally suitable materials with ethnic minority populations have been discussed. Much conventional equipment can be modified to suit the child's culture and interests.

For assessment our usual set-up includes play-house materials: a cooker, saucepans, tea/dinner sets, with additional Asian cooking utensils including steel basins and dishes. A griddle pan is supplied together with a rolling-pin and board and 'playdoh' for making chappatis. Plastic fruit is the other 'food' supplied, as it is universally familiar. Other useful materials include a cot, push-chair, iron and ironing-board. A range of commercially available Asian dolls (with removable clothes) and puppets are also used, together with familiar soft toys — teddy bears, stuffed animals, etc. Older children enjoy miniature dolls' house play, and again, Asian doll families are available. In addition to symbolic play materials, constructional and manipulative toys, such as pull-along telephones, bricks and other stacking toys, Lego, pop-up cone trees, simple formboards, posting boxes, etc., are often familiar and useful in encouraging interaction. Footballs and toy cars, trucks and aeroplanes are also favourites. A range of activities can be elicited by using simple materials such as cardboard boxes, tins, cotton reels, sticks, and so on. Children's books with a suitable ethnic content — particularly those with photographs depicting Asian family life — are also popular.

Assessment procedure

Initially the family is asked to interact naturally with the child during shared play activities, without any interference from the clinicians, who observe from another room. This sample of communication immediately identifies the extent and variety of languages heard, understood and possibly spoken by the child, together with potential areas of difficulty.

Following this initial observation period, the therapists join the family, in order to collect more specific information in identified areas using specially devised assessment materials to augment the spontaneous language sample, such as a phonological word list which includes Panjabi/Urdu phonemes in different word positions, with words chosen for their phonetic possibilities and cultural familiarity. Allowance is made for English versions of words such as 'ball' and 'book', which are very commonly 'borrowed' by Panjabi/Urdu speakers.

In addition to obtaining observed data about the child's communicative functioning in clinic, use is made of a social-communication questionnaire for completion at home or, in possible cases of illiteracy, for verbal administration in the clinic. The questionnaire aims to collect information about the words or phrases used by the child in all languages and in different contexts, and to identify any immature or non-verbal attempts to communicate. The structured format of the questionnaire makes it a particularly useful method of encouraging informative parental reporting and supports the usual information gained from a case history. The additional considerations involved in bilingual case history administration has been covered in detail elsewhere (Miller, 1979).

Initial evaluation of observations takes place during the session and is then discussed between both therapists and family members. More detailed evaluation of the data continues over the assessment period, and again relies on general norms and information from the family. **Receptive language** is evaluated through watching the child's interaction with family members. Early processes, such as auditory attention and selective listening, and understanding of words in context, with or without gesture, can be observed; assessment of more advanced levels of comprehension is more difficult, since it involves greater syntactic, semantic and conceptual complexity, but in practice we find that identification of comprehension difficulties with the pre-school age-group is not always as complicated as it may sound. Processes such as the inability to attend selectively, and particularly to listen accurately, often underlie such difficulties, and can be observed without necessarily analysing linguistic structure.

The **pragmatics** of the child's communication is assessed, as with any monolingual child, through checklists of behaviour in different contexts, and the additional pragmatic area of code differentiation which needs assessing in the bilingual child, can be ascertained through observation and discussion with the family.

Evaluation of **syntactic and semantic** development is achieved through the use of profiles constructed from a language sample, applying the principles behind monolingual assessment procedures such as LARSP, PRISM-G (Crystal et al., 1976; Crystal, 1987) and an estimate of mean length of utterance (MLU) (Chapman, 1981). All utterances are counted and profiled in a combination of languages, if necessary, and comments about language dominance, or about processes such as lexical borrowing, are added. We find that some **phonological** processes can be identified using conventional methods of analysis (Grunwell, 1982), and experience with this group of language-delayed children shows that very similar processes — e.g. stopping, fronting, cluster simplification and reduplication — occur in Panjabi and Urdu, as well as in other languages. This similarity of processes across linguistic boundaries has been noted elsewhere (Ball and Jones, 1984), and means that on a practical level, analysis of processes can lead to a working diagnosis of delay or disorder, despite a lack of normative data. Evaluation of **fluency** is carried out in conventional ways: noting frequency and types of dysfluency in a sample of language, and obtaining comprehensive information from the family. An added dimension is the comparison of fluency in different languages, as well as in different contexts, and for this we rely on information from family members in addition to our own recorded information.

Obviously assessment is a continuing process, but we find the initial assessment period of a pre-school bilingual child often takes longer than usual. It may require several sessions at home, as well as in the other setting.

Management

Following discussion of assessment results and a decision to intervene, language therapy takes the usual form of modelling, discussion and advice about activities to be carried out at home.

For the bilingual, pre-school child management procedures need to be adapted for linguistic, but mainly sociocultural, reasons. Obviously we include the whole family whenever possible, but it has been found that liaison via the most influential family member is of great benefit as this co-ordinates the management process well. Although the ultimate language choice remains with the family, they may require information about the normal process of bilingualism, including details of lexical borrowing, code differentiation, code-switching, and so on. When deciding on activities or objects to be employed in therapy, the family particularly needs to be consulted.

Once appropriate goals, activities and materials have been selected, modelling of the activities is considered to be of the utmost importance, especially in cases where the parents are unfamiliar with the concept of learning through play. Demonstration of tasks involving such things as turn-taking, selective listening or waiting for a verbal signal in the appropriate language, for example, has shown positive results, and the involvement of two therapists at this stage greatly facilitates the process.

When working with a pre-verbal 2½-year-old child, who rarely attended to or understood language, one therapist carried out the activity requiring the child to wait for the word 'go!' before kicking a ball, while the other therapist gave a running commentary of the activity to parents in their mother tongue. This enabled them to observe the activity and its positive effects and, at the same time, to listen to the explanation and ask questions without interruption from the child.

Modelling appropriate language input is almost always carried out in the child's mother tongue, and explained carefully in either English or Panjabi/Urdu. This is often a joint effort. For example, when encouraging reduction of complex language used with a 3-year-old at the single-word stage, one therapist modelled two-element verbal input in Panjabi using culturally appropriate Play-house play with the child, while the other therapist was able to explain, in English, the concept of learning language through play, together with the significance of appropriately modified language input.
Structured tasks, especially those involving materials perceived as 'educational', tend to be more enthusiastically adopted by our families and seem to be more successful than general advice about language development. Again, the mother tongue is mainly the medium of therapy, but this can be modified.

Nadeem, a 2-year-old boy presented with delayed-language development, his attention and listening skills being particularly poor. It had been established that the main language of the home was Panjabi and the four older, school-aged siblings used Panjabi with their parents, but English with one another. Nadeem's mother had found it difficult to follow general suggestions at home, such as simplifying and shortening her sentences, following Nadeem's lead, etc., despite demonstration and some practice of these activities in the clinic. The therapist then modelled a structured activity with Nadeem in Panjabi which involved naming one object, posting it into a box and saying 'gone'. Nadeem responded well to this activity and began to imitate 'gone'. His mother then joined in, and not only carried out the activity accurately, but also simplified her language input in this situation and controlled Nadeem's attention well. The activity was suggested for the home programme, the choice and number of objects having been discussed with Nadeem's mother.

During a subsequent visit home by the clinicians, Nadeem was found sitting in a large box with a hole in the side, posting the objects and spontaneously using 'gone'. The game was extended to include selection of one out of two objects by name, followed by 'gone'. His mother attempted this in Panjabi, and the siblings, who naturally used English with Nadeem, successfully attempted the task in this language. This reinforcement in the second language appeared to help Nadeem without confusing him, and communication for the family members remained natural.

The additional use of video recordings for feedback to parents can be invaluable, for example, in cases where the parents' language input to a child is too complex or where they are over-directing her play. Replay of recordings to parents not only helps them to identify such behaviours in themselves, but also improves their self-monitoring, thereby leading to a more appropriate input.

Therapy programmes and advice leaflets are provided in the mother tongue or English as needed.

Home visits, although time-consuming, do present a true picture of the child within the context of his family and may, in some cases, be the most appropriate environment for therapy.

Hasan, a language-delayed Urdu speaking child was brought to the clinic by both parents. His mother spoke to him in Urdu, while his bilingual father chose to speak English. Appropriate activities to be carried out at home were modelled both in English and Urdu. After two clinic visits Hasan appeared to have made no progress, and it was felt that the parents had not understood the concept underlying therapy. A home visit was felt to be appropriate. Hasan's mother was not only more relaxed at home, but also practised the activities, once these were re-demonstrated, with greater enthusiasm. It later became evident that not only had his mother been inhibited by the unfamiliar clinic situation, but she had also felt unable to play with the child in the presence of her husband. Hasan subsequently made good progress and home therapy appeared to have been a contributory factor.

Not all home visits are equally successful. Distractions encountered, such as overgenerous hospitality, together with large numbers of interested family acquaintances 'dropping in' to view the proceedings has sometimes hindered intervention aims. On these occasions, we derive comfort from the thought that the visits have some information as well as entertainment value.

Evaluation

Nearly half the children seen at the clinic in its first year were referred by speech therapists, the main reasons being the existence of a language barrier between the clinician and family, and the difficulties of obtaining the service of bilingual facilitators. Other referrals received were from paediatricians, medical officers and health visitors. Almost all referrals received were appropriate. The majority of children referred were in the pre-school age-group and 75% of them were passive bilinguals. As anticipated, Panjabi has been found to be the majority L1, Urdu being the L1 for the remaining children.

Involvement of the Panjabi/Urdu speaking clinician has naturally been of benefit for several reasons: the linguistic/cultural barrier normally existing between the family and clinician is overcome; appointment letters and intervention programmes in an appropriate script can be provided; inhibition in the presence of strangers, particularly in the home setting, can be overcome more easily; since the clinician is already trained to assess and treat disorders of communication, compiling a phonological screening-list, writing programmes, transcribing utterances phonetically, etc. is considerably easier than it would be for a bilingual facilitator; and because the clinician has a knowledge of the underlying management principles, counselling of families can be easier.

Difficulties are none the less encountered. While our approach works well for language-delayed children, it may not be adequate in cases of specific language disorder where a more comprehensive linguistic approach may be required. Sometimes there are dialectal differences between the family's and clinician's mother tongue, and sometimes the higher level of lexical borrowing in the clinician's speech requires adjustment. This situation is usually easily resolved by asking family members to monitor the clinician's utterances and to draw her attention to any differences as these arise. Counselling is not necessarily straightforward, since the clinician has been trained in English, and equivalent words or expressions are not always available — a point worth bearing in mind when involving bilingual co-workers.

Despite an ideal appointment system and provision of transport, attendance has not been complete, due partly to sudden departures of the family abroad for unspecified periods, a common occurrence with the British Asian population.

The availability of two clinicians and video equipment is of obvious benefit. One anticipated difficulty was that some Muslim families would object, on religious grounds, to video recordings being made. This has not been encountered to date; the only adjustment occasionally requested has been to keep the camera focused on the child rather than on female members of the family.

We have been unable to overcome the problems of maternal isolation and referral of children to mother-tongue playgroups, since appropriate community-backed provision, including self-help schemes, are not currently available in Manchester for the Pakistani population, although suitable provision for the Bengali and Iranian communities exists. It is hoped that provision will be increased in the near future. Group therapy for some children, with involvement of parents, is another possibility worth considering.

From this experience it appears that setting up of special bilingual clinics can be successful in meeting some of the needs of the pre-school bilingual population, especially when backed up with community support.

CONCLUSION

Young bilingual children are as likely to present with a range of communication delays and disorders as are children in the general population; when considering British Asian pre-schoolers, in particular, the speech therapist can be faced with the need to treat children from different sociocultural backgrounds, who may be exposed to several non-English languages. Even though many of these children can be described as bilingual only in the 'passive' sense, language intervention remains complicated and requires special attention, time and staffing. The increasing number of bilingual speech therapists being trained and employed can only help improve the quality of intervention with this group of children. However, individual bilingual speaking therapists cannot always cover the range and diversity of languages encountered in many speech therapy clinics, and the involvement of bilingual co-workers/interpreters remains necessary. The training of such co-workers, and the training of therapists in the best ways to use their services, is a priority. This provision, together with the kind of modifications to the content and process of intervention which are suggested above in the description of a special bilingual clinic, makes it possible successfully to identify and remediate communication problems in bilingual children at a suitably early age. It is hoped that this early intervention will reduce the number of children having to struggle with the additional majority language on entering school, at a stage when their L1 is still severely delayed or disordered.

10

The Bilingual Child with Special Educational Needs

Angela Roberts and Dorothy A. Gibbs

INTRODUCTION

The bilingually language handicapped child who has additional special educational needs is the focus of this chapter. The legislative climate and the range of service provision for bilingual (and potentially so) children at different ages and with different needs is covered. The issues involved with the pre-schooler with special needs are discussed and home teaching services reviewed. The issues in the management of the older bilingual child in special education are discussed, as well as the alternative and augmentative systems of communication available.

The main emphasis of the chapter rests on the special needs of physical and slow-learning handicaps which are involved with language-learning problems; however, visual and hearing impairments are also referred to.

Finally, the importance of inter-professional liaison is discussed throughout the chapter and is specifically illustrated by discussion of the role of a special-needs liaison worker (SNLW).

THE 1981 EDUCATION ACT (ENGLAND, WALES AND NORTHERN IRELAND)

With the arrival of the *Education Act 1981,* children under age 2 who may have special needs can be assessed with the consent of (or at the request of) their parents. The 1981 Act, with application to children with special needs in England, Wales and Northern Ireland, has given parents the right to obtain mainstream education (with adequate resources) for children with special needs. As far as the non-English speaking population is concerned, the Act states that: 'A child is not to be taken as having a learning difficulty solely because the language (or form of the language) in which he is or will be taught is different from a language (or form of the language) which has at any time been spoken in his home.' The Act further states that any English as a Second Language (ESL) pupil thought to be in need of special education *must* be assessed by an expert who knows the language of her home.

In the USA the Public Law also recognizes the issues affecting assessments of bilingual children and states that: 'The assessment of a handicapped child is to be carried out through the child's native language.'

SERVICE PROVISION AND FAMILY NEEDS

With advances in the detection and early identification of children with certain handicapping conditions, service providers can become involved at an early stage. In response to the growing awareness of the need for early and continued involvement with these children and their families, provision for the handicapped child often begins long before the issue of school placement has been resolved.

Provision for children with special needs varies from area to area, depending on the services available, and may take various forms, including attendance at a multidisciplinary assessment unit, or participation in some visiting teacher or home teaching programme, such as the Portage scheme, prior to placement in a special school or unit.

According to McGown (1982), the needs of families with a handicapped child vary, and the way in which parents cope with a handicapped child is dependent on a number of factors, including their level of personal understanding, their attitudes and resources, emotional, physical and financial, and the support they receive from other family members, neighbours and all professional advisers. As McGown states, 'children with handicaps must be considered within the context of their families and each family with a handicapped child needs individual consideration' (p. 292).

With these last points particularly in mind, it is the purpose of the following discussion to highlight a few of the many issues which warrant careful consideration when attempting to work with children with special needs who come from families where English is not the first language.

ISSUES ARISING INITIALLY DURING THE EARLY PRE-SCHOOL PERIOD

Powell and Perkins's (1984) study of Asian families with a preschool handicapped child, living in some of Birmingham's inner city areas, explored the extent to which such families could benefit from help in teaching their children new skills, and elicited from these families some indication of the resources they felt they needed to help them bring up their handicapped child.

The main finding of this study was that the families interviewed demonstrated a real lack of knowledge of their child's handicap and of the services available to them. Basic information about the nature of the handicap had not been assimilated by parents — or it had not been given to them.

Most parents wanted advice about teaching their child new skills, and the study showed that the families needed a person fluent in their mother tongue to help them make use of existing services and to enable the services to become more useful to the families.

The importance of effective communication between families of children with special needs and service providers cannot be over-emphasized, at any stage, but perhaps the period when this is particularly crucial is during the early stages of the child's development, starting from the point when the child's special needs are first identified or suspected.

Although the general aim for successful communication will not differ when dealing with children from English speaking and ethnolinguistic backgrounds, there are additional challenges to be overcome when dealing with families whose primary language differs from that of the therapist or other service providers.

Much of the success of attempts at early intervention with such families lies in the availability of experienced bilingual co-workers who are fluent in the family's mother tongue and familiar with the cultures from which the families come.

Baby Kauser was referred to the hospital speech therapist within the first 2 days of life because she was found to have a cleft palate. This is a condition in which the roof of the mouth fails to develop normally during the early stages of intra-uterine life, and which can give rise to feeding and speech problems which will be of particular concern to the speech therapist as the child develops.

Without the services of the bilingual co-worker, it would have been impossible to convey to the mother the reason for the speech therapist's presence at the baby's feeding times during those early days, or to outline the role that the speech therapist would play, and the types of problems she might be able to offer help with during the coming months and years.

When attempting to work with children from bilingual backgrounds who have special needs, it is essential to be aware of and sensitive to cultural differences in attitudes, ideas and priorities which may exist in these families, and which may have a significant effect on the outcome of any proposed therapy or teaching programme.

Take, for example, the complex and often sensitive area of developing appropriate feeding skills in the infant and young child with physical difficulties and/or learning difficulties. The development of feeding is important for a number of reasons:

1. As a means of obtaining sufficient nourishment for life;
2. As an important social skill;
3. As a preparation for the later development of speech.

The child with a physical problem, or a child with severe learning difficulties, may experience feeding difficulties, the nature and severity of which are often dependent on the extent of the child's overall difficulties. These feeding difficulties often become a source of great anxiety and distress to parents and family.

It is important that these children and their families receive early and continued help to enable them to progress, within their limited capabilities, through the stages of feeding, and to avoid unduly prolonged delay at any of the early stages in the developmental sequence. Such delay may adversely affect later speech development.

When attempting to intervene in the management of feeding skills, it is essential to appreciate the circumstances existing within the home environment and to approach remediation and management with an awareness of the effect that cultural differences in areas such as child-rearing practices may have on the success of the intended programme.

Working together with a bilingual co-worker when discussing with mothers issues involved in the management of feeding their handicapped or developmentally delayed children has proved invaluable. This is another area which would be extremely difficult, if not impossible, for the monolingual therapist to tackle without such support.

HOME TEACHING SERVICES

In response to the growing awareness of the need for early and continued involvement with children with special needs and their families, the number of pre-school intervention services, in which parents are shown how to help their child acquire new skills, is increasing rapidly.

Evidence suggests that home teaching services, such as Portage, in which families of pre-school handicapped children are visited in their homes on a regular weekly basis and shown how to teach their children selected new skills, can be successfully delivered to Asian families. However, if such a service is to be successful, workers need to be sensitive to possible different attitudes, ideas and priorities of the families involved (Bardsley and Perkins, 1983). This study presents information about the outcome of the Portage scheme with Asian families in central Birmingham, and suggests that while such a scheme can be effective, qualitative differences exist in the service delivery to Asian and monolingual English families. These differences were thought to be due, perhaps, to the effect of differences in child-rearing practices, differing attitudes towards and opportunities for play within the home and differing reactions to handicap among the Asian families. Activities such as play are not regarded as adult activities, nor are they seen as learning activities, so careful planning and explanation of such activities is necessary.

Powell and Perkins (1984) investigated the possibility of using a home teaching programme, such as Portage, with Asian families with a handicapped child. They established four important factors which are likely to influence the outcome of such a programme:

1. Belief in child development;
2. Belief in teaching;
3. Knowledge of handicap;
4. Opportunities for teaching.

Lack of information and various religious beliefs often stop parents from participating in their child's early development. However, these can be overcome by setting activities that parents are happy to attempt. Play activities can be extremely productive when initiated by the child's older siblings. Certain teaching techniques might have to be introduced and demonstrated by the Portage worker, for example, the use of reinforcers such as praise and smiles for successful attempts at the required tasks and for good behaviour.

ISSUES AFFECTING THE DEVELOPMENT OF COMMUNICATION SKILLS IN BILINGUAL CHILDREN WITH SPECIAL NEEDS

As has already been mentioned in this and other chapters of this book, assessment of a child's mother-tongue language acquisition, in addition to an assessment of the extent of second language development, is essential if the most appropriate form of remediation is to be provided. This is particularly relevant when discussing children who have physical disabilities and/or learning difficulties as it is widely accepted that children having such problems are more likely to have language problems than their non-handicapped peers.

Without this effort to obtain information about both L1 and L2 language development, one cannot begin to draw any conclusions as to whether the presenting language problems are of a general language-learning nature, or of a more specific type of problem in learning English as a second language. As detailed discussion of the assessment of L1 and L2 language development has already been undertaken in this book, a number of other issues connected with the development of communication skills in the bilingual child with special needs will now be discussed.

ASSOCIATED SENSORY DEFECTS

Often children with physical problems due to central nervous system impairment can, and do, have associated sensory defects, which contribute to their language reception and acquisition problems. Early detection and remediation of the difficulties whenever possible is essential if long-lasting problems are to be minimized.

However, for some families from non-English speaking households, attendance at clinic and hospital appointments can be a significant problem due to communication difficulties involved. Delay in detection and treatment of these sensory problems can sometimes occur due to failed appointments, but hopefully with close liaison between home, school and ethnic support and medical services involved, such delays can be kept to a minimum.

Once prostheses, such as hearing aids or glasses, have been prescribed, further problems occur in their maintenance and use. These arise from communication difficulties and misunderstandings between the professionals supplying the appliance and the family and school. For example, two pairs of glasses may need to be obtained for one child to ensure that she has a pair for school use. Correct hearing-aid cleaning and maintenance can be another problem area. These misunderstandings can be resolved or avoided by careful discussion of the issues involved with the family, through the bilingual co-worker.

Despite ensuring that every measure is taken to minimize the handicapping effect of sensory and other defects, some children with severe physical and learning disabilities are unable to develop intelligible speech. These children need to acquire or be provided with some other form of communication at the earliest possible stage.

ALTERNATIVE OR AUGMENTATIVE SYSTEMS OF COMMUNICATION

A number of alternative or augmentative systems are now available using signs or symbols, and it is important that through careful assessment of a number of important areas, the most suitable means of communication is selected. With the tremendous advances in recent years in the use and application of technology with the handicapped, it is possible for even the most severely handicapped child to be provided with a means of communication if only at a very basic level. A variety of factors need to be taken into account and given careful consideration before any decision to introduce an alternative or augmentative system of communication can be made.

Many of the issues surrounding the introduction of such a system are likely to be similar when dealing with a monolingual English speaking family, and a family from an ethnolinguistic background. The crucial factor in the success of any such project with a bilingual family would appear to lie in the involvement of, and communication with, the child's immediate family, and close liaison between involved professionals from health and education and the individual's parents and carers through a person fluent in the family's mother tongue. Prior to the introduction of any communication system and throughout the planning, development and implementation phases of the programme, discussion and consultation with all relevant personnel is essential if any measure of success is to be achieved.

Success in this area, with both bilingual and monolingual English speaking families rests largely on their support for, and understanding of, their child's need for a communication system other than a verbal one. This is a complex area, and one which needs to be tackled at an early stage. During such discussions a number of issues need to be raised, for example, the parental view of the child's present level of language development and expectations for the future, parents' understanding of the long-term implications of the child's handicap and their views regarding the communication needs of their child within the home situation. Their knowledge of, and attitudes towards, non-verbal means of communication need to be carefully evaluated during these early discussions.

Assuming the decision to introduce an alternative or augmentative system of communication is taken, family members should be consulted and their views sought where appropriate about the most suitable form of system to be introduced, and its composition.

Picture communication charts

If the child is at a very early stage in developing communication skills, it may be appropriate to provide a picture communication chart, assuming the child has reached the stage where she can recognize pictorial material. Such a communication chart would consist of a small number of pictures (e.g. food, drink, toilet) which would enable the child to make her basic needs known.

Once the decision to provide a communication chart has been made, the child's family should be included in the selection of pictures to be included on the chart. In addition, the child is provided with a chart for home use.

For the child with greater ability and more complex communication needs a number of graphic symbol systems exist. These can be displayed in various ways and accessed by means of finger or eye pointing, or in the case of the severely physically handicapped child, by using electronic devices. One such symbol system, which would appear to be particularly applicable for use with children from dual language backgrounds, is the Blissymbol system.

The Blissymbol system

The Blissymbol system consists of a large number of visual symbols, which can be combined and displayed in various ways to provide a total means of communication, or to augment existing/developing expressive skills. The system is logical and easy to follow, as the symbols are meaning-referenced and can be interpreted without reference to sounds or words. For those unfamiliar with the system each symbol, displayed on a chart, can be accompanied by an appropriate written word (the Blissymbol system is discussed more fully in McDonald, 1982; Bailey and Jenkinson, 1976 and Galloway, 1978). Blissymbols are used in more than 35 countries, including Israel, French and English speaking regions of Canada, and India, where a large number of languages and dialects are spoken.

Each Blissymbol chart can be constructed to meet the personal communication needs of the user. To aid communication between professionals, the child and the family, and to help bridge the language barriers which may exist, symbols on the chart can be accompanied by the written words of all languages/dialects used within home and school environments. This feature of the Blissymbol system, that is its ability to provide a means of communication, which goes beyond all language barriers, would seem to make it an especially attractive tool for clinicians working with children with special needs from ethnolinguistic backgrounds.

The Blissymbol system can be used with children with limited cognitive abilities or severe language learning difficulties, or with children whose receptive language is developing normally and whose difficulties are restricted to the expressive modality. In the former group symbols are often used to communicate most basic needs, and children may acquire only a small number of symbols which they use individually, or combine to form simple units. Children in the latter group may acquire a large symbol vocabulary, which can be used to produce various sentences. In these cases careful consideration needs to be given to the layout of the symbols on the chart, particularly if the system is to be used in more than one linguistic environment.

In commercially available symbol charts, symbols are arranged in columns according to their grammatical form, and in such a way as to allow for the production of syntactically correct sentences. However, the Blissymbol system allows charts to be personalized in order to meet the particular needs of the individual child.

For instance, in cases where the system is to be used in more than one linguistic context, careful thought should be given to the layout of symbols on the chart, taking into account the form and structure of the languages involved, and the levels of language to be used in each context. Perhaps it would be appropriate to provide two (or more) charts in such cases. For example, one chart could have words written underneath the symbols in the language of that particular environment, and the child could be offered a chart for each of her linguistic environments.

As with all augmentative or alternative forms of communication, successful introduction depends largely on the involvement and support of the Blissymbol user's family at all stages of the system's introduction and use.

Electronic aids

It has been mentioned earlier that advances in the application of technology in meeting the needs of the handicapped have enabled even the severely handicapped to have some means of communication. These advances in the availability and design of electronic aids and communication systems raises some interesting issues when considering children growing up in dual or multi-language environments. Technology now exists to produce personalized communication systems to meet the individual needs of the user, and to provide a range of means for accessing symbol systems such as Bliss. A growing number of electronic aids incorporate some form of speech output, which adds a new dimension to the usefulness of the aid in communicating situations.

As the facility exists (though not yet widely available) to make the synthetic voice of the communication aid similar to that of the user in terms of gender, age and local dialect, special consideration has to be given to these factors when developing a system for a bilingual child. Should the system be produced to facilitate communication primarily within the educational environment, and if so, what effect will this have on the child's communication and interaction within the home environment? Consultation with the child's family in discussions about design features of such a system is important as these features may ultimately determine the acceptance and long-term success of the communication aid.

Perhaps the time will come when electronic communication aids with speech facilities will be able to overcome the additional challenges arising with children from dual language backgrounds?

The family have a central role to play in the selection of a vocabulary to be included in their child's communication system. It is not sufficient to base a communication system upon only the assessment of the child's needs during the school day. A detailed knowledge of the child's personal home circumstances, and communication needs within that context, is an essential prerequisite to vocabulary selection and display. This is borne out further in implementing the Makaton Vocabulary.

The Makaton Vocabulary

The Makaton Vocabulary, originally begun as a project to teach sign language to deaf, mentally handicapped adults, is now widely used in its revised form with children and adults with learning difficulties. It is also used with other language handicapped people.

Makaton was designed to provide a controlled method of teaching a specific developmental vocabulary of signs from British Sign Language (BSL), in order to provide a basic means of communication (Walker, 1978; Walker and Armfield, 1981).

The signs can be used to bridge the gaps between two languages, and parents and family members need to be taught the signs. The purpose of Makaton must always be fully explained —

i.e. for some it will be used to provide a basic means of communication, while for others it will be used to facilitate natural speech and language development. Makaton signs can be used with other language labels such as Panjabi, Bengali and Turkish. The signs should always be accompanied by normal grammatical speech; and the signs should be presented in the same basic order as the spoken language.

Margaret Walker, founder of the Makaton Programme, has modified the programme to include signs which are useful and unique for different cultures. Makaton also serves as a useful link between school and home where parents can communicate with the child about school activities.

The following case study highlights some of the issues discussed earlier in connection with working with the bilingual child with special needs and the family. It is intended to show how more careful attention to some of the particular problems involved might lead to the provision of a communication system of greater functional value to the child, carers and those in the child's school environment.

Zafar was the fourth of seven children from a Panjabi speaking family. He had been diagnosed as having cerebral palsy at an early age, and at the age of 7 was now wheelchair-bound and reliant on his family to meet even his most basic needs. One of his younger siblings had similar motor problems.

Zafar's verbal communication skills were significantly impaired, with receptive (comprehension) skills far in advance of expressive capabilities. Expressive skills, in English, were limited to a small number of single words which were not used spontaneously, but could be illicited during individual language sessions.

Through informal mother-tongue language assessment, and family reports, it was apparent that Zafar's communication problems crossed language boundaries, and skills appeared to be at a similar level in both languages. In view of Zafar's limited expressive skills, in the presence of relatively intact comprehension, it was decided by school staff that an augmentative system of communication should be introduced. The Blissymbol system was felt to be most appropriate in this case as Zafar had previously demonstrated good picture/drawing recognition, and although physical limitations made any manual signing system impractical, he was able to point with reasonable accuracy to symbols on a board.

A small 'core' vocabulary of symbols, which had a high degree of functional value in the school environment was selected, and a structured school-based programme of symbol introduction and instruction was undertaken with Zafar.

During these very early stages of symbol introduction/ selection contact with Zafar's family took the form of a number of home visits by a member of the team involved in the symbol work in school. Unfortunately, these visits were carried out without the assistance of any bilingual co-worker, and all communication took place with two sisters who played a major role in caring for Zafar and his handicapped younger sister.

It soon became clear that Zafar's family had little idea of the long-term nature and implications of his motor problems and associated difficulties (including communication difficulties); and they had a very limited understanding of his communication needs in view of these difficulties. Also it became clear that Zafar's communication needs in the home were in fact totally different from those that had been envisaged by staff in the school setting. A number of symbols which had been selected as being of great importance were redundant and of little value to Zafar once consideration was given to the communication demands made on him at home. This may well have accounted, in part, for Zafar's reluctance to use the chart spontaneously to initiate communication, despite his obvious ability to learn the symbol meanings and to use them in response to questions during structured sessions.

Clearly, if the introduction of a communication system was to have any long-term benefit for Zafar, his family and his school, much closer contact and involvement with the family both in the programme planning and execution of the system was needed. Detailed discussion of the long-term implications of Zafar's difficulties, and the purpose of introducing a symbol system, was seen to be crucial. This type of discussion could only be achieved with the assistance of a bilingual co-worker fluent in the home language, and familiar with the principles of introducing augmentative systems of communication. Indeed, at all stages of introducing such a system to a bilingual child and family a co-worker of this type is an essential ingredient for success.

School-based speech and language programmes

In the school setting articulation work also forms a part of the speech and language programme. Once the child has enough language skills to communicate, it is useful to begin work on the child's articulation, if that is felt to be required. However, it is important that all members of staff are kept informed at every stage in the articulation programme.

As with monolingual children, bilingual children with special needs require frequent repetition and reinforcement. They can benefit from specialized teaching techniques and programmes.

The Derbyshire Language Scheme

The Derbyshire Language Scheme is a system of language teaching aimed at improving the language skills of children, whose development in this area is delayed. The scheme, originally developed as part of the curriculum of a school for children with severe learning difficulties, grew directly from the needs of the children involved. Based on a knowledge of normal language acquisition, the scheme places particular emphasis on the teaching of language skills necessary for everyday life.

Bearing in mind some of its practical and theoretical limitations, the scheme is a useful programme. It is flexible regarding the materials used and does not dictate a specific method of teaching. Parents, family members and teachers may all become involved in the child's programme.

The scheme, which offers a wide range of activities for developing receptive and expressive language skills, is divided into a number of stages. At the lowest levels, the child is introduced to the idea of communicating using gestures, sounds and eventually words. Once single words emerge, the activities attempt to move the child on to two-word combinations and then sentences containing three, four and five words in a series of carefully graded steps. The more complex sections of the scheme focus the child's attention on various aspects of grammar and complex sentence formation.

The first two stages of the scheme, in which understanding and expression of single-word and two-word utterances is attempted, are similar in English and other languages such as Panjabi or Bengali. At this level noun–noun and noun–verb combinations in these languages have the same word order. Such similarities should be used positively to gain parents' confidence in teaching their children. In later stages one would have to be careful about the word order and the number of information-carrying words in any selected structure. If the scheme's format is to be used to develop skills in languages other than English, the word order of languages such as Panjabi and Bengali which are different from English, must be taken into account.

THE VISUALLY AND HEARING IMPAIRED

The discussion of alternative and augmentative communication systems similarly applies when working with bilingual children who have visual and hearing impairments. For the visually impaired child who comes from a bilingual community the production of braille in the scripts of other languages, as for Panjabi-Gurmuki in the UK, goes some way to bridging the culture/communication gap. Certainly, this area needs more investigation and resources.

The issues involved in the use of Makaton Vocabulary become rather more fraught when using sign language with the hearing impaired child from a bilingual community. British Sign Language (BSL) and its American counterpart are based on signed English. It seems necessary to develop signed languages for other languages, too. Whether these sign languages would be unique, or modified versions of BSL, would require investigation. Practitioners and parents would need to learn these sign languages in order to offer language choice to the signing/hearing impaired child from a bilingual community. Since many signing/hearing impaired children develop their own inter-community sign language and are consequently 'diglossic', offering further signed language choice cannot be ruled out of hand. Debate will continue as to the advisability and efficacy of such a communication strategy, and here resources and research would be well spent.

So far in this chapter we have dealt primarily with the role of the speech therapist in the multi-disciplinary team. The following section describes the role of an educationally funded liaison teacher in this team. It is an example of how one education authority chose to organize more effectively its management of the bilingually language-impaired child with additional special needs.

THE ROLE OF THE SPECIAL-NEEDS LIAISON WORKER

In 1980, Sandwell, a local education authority in the West Midlands, bordering Birmingham, established a post of special-needs liaison worker (SNLW) within its Ethnic Minorities Support Service. The brief for this post holder is to be responsible for the individual school-aged ethnic minority child with a learning, physical, emotional or social problem. Its aims are to provide a multi-agency approach to facilitate diagnosis and treatment, and to develop and sustain links between the home, school and agencies involved with the care of the child and her family. The task is often a detective assignment.

For example, when the ethnic minority pupil presents with a learning problem, several explanations are possible. She may be simply limited by her lack of listening/speaking/reading/writing skills in English. She could have a specific reading difficulty which is, or would be, present in her first language as well, or she could have a language disability which inhibits her oral acquisition of *any* language. Her learning problem may be due to sensory difficulties which inhibit her visual or aural apprehension of language. She may have overall low ability.

If hearing loss is suspected, who will give instruction for a pure sound test in Panjabi, Arabic or Pushto! Who has a chart for testing vision with Chinese characters, or who can ask questions about the symbols in Bengali? If global difficulties or specific learning disabilities are considered probable, who has intelligence or perceptual tests in Urdu or Gujerati and the training to administer them?

The tools and personnel for differential diagnosis in languages other than English seem to be in short supply in English speaking countries. Bruck (1984) notes the possible consequence of this deficiency. Writing of consideration for the education of Canadian children with specific learning difficulties, she highlights the situation which often occurs. Referring to studies by Damico, Oller and Storey (1981), Mercer (1973) and Cummins (1980), she points out that 'methods for diagnosis and treatment of learning disabilities for the middle-class Anglophone child are much more straightforward than for the child schooled in a second language and/or from a minority background' (p. 124). This lack of appropriate tools and methods can lead to either one of two unsatisfactory results, as Bruck suggests. Many minority children are diagnosed as 'handicapped' when their primary difficulties lie in inadequate knowledge of the school language and/or the middle-class educational culture. Therefore, professionals may err on the side of caution and fail to recognize actual difficulties. As Bruck suggests, 'since there are at present, no reliable or valid instruments to assess the primary problems of minority background children, there is reluctance to attribute school failure to inherent psychological characteristics (e.g. low IQ, learning disability, etc.) of the minority child' (p. 12).

Consequently, the ethnic minority child often does not receive appropriate help. As Bruck states, 'By avoiding proper identification, educators are actually preventing the minority child from receiving adequate treatment for his or her problems' (pp. 124–5).

Case excerpts

The following cases should provide samples of the range of difficulties encountered in catering for the special needs of school-aged ethnic minority children.

> Nadeem was referred to the SNLW by a teacher on the remedial and advisory team of the Child Psychology Service. At age 8 years he was having great difficulty in copying an oral or written model. Granted, he had only been back in England for six months after four years in Pakistan, but he did not seem to respond as other beginners. Informal Panjabi assessment using a checklist for syntax compiled by a speech therapist and a Panjabi teacher showed comprehension and expression only of two-element structures, of the 'man sit' variety. Nadeem could use only the verb root, with no inflections for number, gender or tense. A visit to his father revealed that he had made no progress in the acquisition of English during a year in a West Bromwich nursery, and no progress in the development of his mother tongue during four years in school in Pakistan. Eventually it was concluded that Nadeem's non-verbal skills were equally delayed and he was placed in an ESN(M) school. His mother-tongue development was monitored over the years and showed gradual progress, as did his English under the management of a speech therapist.

> Arfan at age 7 years exhibited a very similar profile as had

Nadeem on assessment of his Panjabi and English language (with the Wheldall Sentence Comprehension Test, revised bilingual version (1987), and the Sandwell Diagnostic Expressive Language Assessment). Both mother tongue and English showed receptive and expressive control only of two-element structures. He was referred by his speech therapist because of his delay in language acquisition, but his teacher pointed out that his number work was excellent. After much confusion and delay, Arfan was eventually found to have binaural hearing loss of 60 dc. When fitted with hearing aids, he began to acquire language at a much faster rate, although he still had quite pronounced phonological difficulties. Furthermore, there were continuing obstacles to communication between the school and medical personnel and Arfan's family, resulting in problems about the care of his aids. It took some time for staff to discover when they were blocked with dirt or broken. The education department was thus faced with making a placement decision which would be the most beneficial to Arfan in light of all his circumstances. Should he be left in the first-year junior mainstream class, where his progress had improved after his aids were fitted, but where he was still lagging substantially behind his peers in language-related subjects, despite assumed good overall abilities? Could his attendance at the Local Speech Therapy Clinic be relied on if this course were followed? Instead, should Arfan be placed in a partially hearing unit where the functioning of his aids could be checked and a weekly visit from a speech therapist be more or less guaranteed? This was the course of action recommended by the ENT consultant in charge. But was segregation from his local peers justified on educational grounds? The course of action adopted in the first instance was for Arfan to remain in his neighbourhood school, but to be brought by an education department taxi to a health centre for bilingual language remediation on two mornings a week (see Chapter 11).

Kashmir presented with a similar picture, with regard to her Panjabi and English language acquisition. The headteacher of her infant school referred her because she was puzzled by Kashmir's lack of oral fluency in English, as opposed to the excellence of her reading. She was considered to be the 'best reader' in her top infant class. It took considerable probing to discover that her comprehension of what she read was quite weak, despite her well-developed work-attack skills. A visit to her home revealed that she had not begun to talk at all until the age of 3 years and that her parents were quite aware of her delayed development of mother tongue. She was referred to the speech therapist at her local clinic because of her expressive language handicap, with mild associated receptive difficulties (Sandwell Diagnostic Expressive Language Assessments, and Wheldall Sentence Comprehension Test, revised bilingual version.)

The overwhelming majority, probably on average 80% of the 80 cases a term attended to by the special-needs liaison worker, are referred for learning or language-learning difficulties. For these children receptive and expressive language assessments in mother tongue and English are a first line of approach. Home visits by the SNLW and a colleague sharing the child's home language to gain insight and developmental information are another basic strategy.

These strategies are often employed as well in cases where emotional or behaviour difficulties are primary. Jatinder, at age 6, was on the 'current' list of a wide range of agencies in the health, education and social services department.

He was being seen by a speech therapist for lack of language development and a child psychiatrist from the Sandwell Young People and Parents' Advisory Service because of his disturbed behaviour. He had been referred to the educational psychologist for lack of progress at school, the audiologist because he appeared not to hear/heed and the social services, educational welfare office and home–school links officer for ethnic minorities to investigate the home situation. Jatinder's acquisition of English was very slight, basically only 'naming', despite a reasonable amount of exposure in his home. However, informal assessment of his Panjabi showed satisfactory syntactic development and adequate use of expressive language when he chose to speak. Jatinder's behaviour was such as to preclude any type of formal assessment procedures. It was hypothesized that language learning was not primary among his difficulties.

Meanwhile, Jatinder's behaviour was deteriorating rapidly. He was destroying plants, continually attacking other children and damaging their work and increasingly putting the safety of himself and other children at risk. At home he threw his baby cousin out of the pram. Further investigation of his situation by the Panjabi speaking home–school links officer revealed a horrifying tale. Jatinder's mother's marriage had been arranged in India with his severely educationally subnormal father who was in England. After three years, she left her husband and moved into a flat, where she later committed suicide in 2-year-old Jatinder's presence; the toddler was left alone with her body for several days before they were discovered. He was at the time of referral primarily in the care of his grandmother, who was fairly frail and lacked control of him. Also present in the home were his grandfather and his aunt and uncle and their three children, of whom Jatinder was intensely, and understandably, jealous. The adults seemed to feel a sense of duty towards him, but little affection.

The agencies concerned were contacted and their efforts co-ordinated. The child-psychiatrist referred him to a residential psychiatric clinic with a small school attached, where full medical, as well as clinical and educational psychological assessments, were carried out. He was found to have some specific learning difficulties, in addition to emotional problems. After six months there, he was placed in a special school in the area where his family lived and where specialized ESL help was available.

Hopefully, this rather lengthy anecdote points up the great number of false assumptions that are possible when making contact with a child and family solely in their second language. Not only can wrong conclusions be drawn about the nature of a child's language acquisition difficulties, but insights into their possible cause(s) are not available. Hence both diagnosis and treatment are drastically hampered, in this case to the point of total non-effectiveness.

In dealing with referrals of bilingual children with physical handicap the problem is not so much in discovering whether language disability is primary as finding out to what extent the primary handicap has affected the language acquisition and development. To this end, the speech therapist in conjunction with the headteacher requested mother-tongue assessments of every Asian pupil who attended the school for the physically handicapped in Sandwell. The results were interesting. In some cases, a very similar profile on the Sandwell Diagnostic Expressive

Language Assessment was obtained in Panjabi as in English. However, for a fairly large number of bilingual pupils, particularly those with central nervous system involvement, the profiles showed considerably more development in English than in the mother tongue. A possible explanation for this pattern could be that children with these difficulties need structured intervention and language support, which they had been receiving for several years in English from the speech therapist and teachers. By contrast, their Panjabi had been left to natural acquisition processes which had exhibited delay. On the other hand, a small number of pupils had Panjabi syntactical profiles which compared favourably with those of their non-handicapped peers, while show-ing little progress in their acquisition of English. On the whole, profiles in both languages were weak in varying degrees as compared to their non-handicapped bilingual peers, some grossly so. But experience suggested caution in predicting potential from assessment at any given time.

> Jagdish, a hydrocephalic boy, was not assessable at age 6 years. He possessed only a handful of formulaic 'Cocktail Party syndrome' phrases which he seemed unable to apply in any meaningful way. When he said 'Sit down', it was just good luck if there were a chair in the vicinity! However, somewhat sur-prisingly, by the age of 7 years he was not only able to cope with the Sandwell Diagnostic Expressive Language Assessment in English and Panjabi, but his total scores were only −1 standard deviation from the mean of his peers and only one or two responses on each scale had to be marked in the 'irrelevant' or 'inappropriate' column. At this point, he joined an ESL group and began to make good progress.

COUNSELLING

The importance of conveying information to, and discussing issues regularly with, parents and relatives of bilingual children with special needs has been stressed throughout this chapter. Despite its obvious significance to the outcome of any service programme, it seems to be an area which is inadequately dealt with in many instances.

Those attempting to take on any form of counselling role should be aware of the presence of language differences and attempt to bridge any communication gap, by means of experienced bilingual co-workers. Issues should be approached with sensitivity and with an awareness of religious and cultural beliefs which may prove to be powerful influencing factors with family members.

Support groups should be encouraged wherever possible, when mothers of the same ethnolinguistic/cultural group can meet together and discuss relevant issues concerning ways of meeting the needs of their handicapped children, and of obtaining best use of the services available to them.

CONCLUSION

In this chapter we have discussed the various aspects of special educational need and the resources which can be made available to meet them. The additional issues concerning the handicapped child from a bilingual community centre on language and culture. The need for appropriate bilingual and bicultural personnel to be involved in the special-needs interdisciplinary team has been clearly illustrated. The importance of this issue lies in the fact that the language and communication of the handicapped child must be developed, particularly in the language of the community who will most probably care most — both emotionally and temporally — for the child. Coming to terms with the handicap has a cultural dimension; consequently, counselling and achieving an understanding of the handicap, its remediation and care may be best effected through the community language of the family.

11

Mainstream Bilingual Schoolchildren: A Model for Remediation

Deirdre M. Duncan and Dorothy A. Gibbs

INTRODUCTION

The model for remediation which is described in this chapter is for group therapy with bilingual children in mainstream education, with language-acquisition problems in both of their languages. The children described are aged between 6 and 9 years, but the remediation model could be used with children of other ages, where appropriate linguistic assessment was carried out in both languages. The children suitable for this therapy arrangement would also be candidates for language units, and this issue is mentioned later (p. 187).

The chapter discusses the challenges presented by the bilingually language handicapped child and the rationale for group therapy, taking up the issue of bilingual therapy. Finally, an example is offered of a model for therapy as practised in the UK in one area of the Midlands with bilingually language handicapped children.

CHALLENGES FOR MANAGEMENT

Referrals

The problem with bilingual language handicap is that it is difficult to detect. There are several reasons for this. Often the child can cope with non-verbal tasks, and a child who speaks very seldom

176

can be thought to have normally developing additional language skills. In minority communities where the first language is part of the culture of that community and is different from the majority community, for example, Asian communities in the UK, Turkish communities in Germany and Austria, or Hispanic communities in the USA, then parents may be reluctant to bring their non-talking children forward for further investigation. Their reluctance could stem from a failure to recognize delay in the child's langue development. It could also stem from the awareness of slight provision and resources for their first language in the majority community.

Another reason for low detection and referral is the prevailing view of language handicap. Children who present with sensory deficits, physical handicap or learning problems are readily recognized as having special needs. Language handicap may be regarded as a 'soft' handicap. That is to say, that the needs of language handicapped people are not so easily recognized, so that they seem to be able to cope with normal living. The degree of non-achievement, failure and disability which language handicap provokes is often obscured. This is even more acute for the child from the bilingual community with language handicap. For these reasons and others (e.g. reluctance to provide resources); provision in the UK for the bilingually language handicapped child is underdeveloped. Indeed, for the English monolingual language handicapped child special-needs provision is very limited.

Language handicap

As with monolingual children, expressive language handicap in bilinguals can manifest itself at a phonological, syntactic, semantic or pragmatic level — often it affects all or a combination of them. This means that children's ability to handle the systems of language is misfunctioning. They cannot grasp the systems of sounds or grammatical structure, or the system of meanings at word or sentence level, or the system of conversational turn-taking and language functions.

Language handicap may be associated with (or be a consequence of) a more major problem, for example, hearing impairment, physical handicap or slow learning. However, there are children who do not have any other identifiable problem and who present with expressive language handicap only.

177

Comprehension of language (receptive language) may also be affected, along with expressive language handicap. Comprehension needs close assessment, which is often very difficult to achieve with children for whom English is a second language because of lack of appropriate assessment procedures and materials.

The children

What are the characteristics of these mainstream school-aged children from bilingual communities which need to be taken into account in considering the assessment and treatment of their language difficulties?

First, we can presume that these children are having a substantial amount of exposure to at least two languages, unlike their pre-school counterparts who may well have daily input only in the mother tongue. By the time a child has spent a year at a primary school, it is possible to gain clues from the rate and pattern of her acquisition of English as a second language (L2) as to whether she has a disability in language learning. Studies (Dulay and Burt, 1977 and Krashen 1978) show that basic morphology and phrase-level structures of L2 English require about 18 months to develop in the normal bilingual child in an English speaking environment. Therefore, if children from linguistic minority communities present after two years of school, having failed to establish basic early-acquired features of English, a strong suspicion of language handicap can be entertained. Obviously the first line of approach would be mother-tongue assessment to confirm that a genuine language-learning difficulty exists. But diagnosis through second language English can also yield valuable information. Furthermore, therapy in English will be useful and necessary in addition to mother-tongue remediation.

Secondly, affective variables (see the Affective Filter Hypothesis in Chapter 2) are a more potent force in the life and development of children of school age than at earlier stages. Many of their energies become engaged in seeking peer interaction, attention and approval, which can provide strong motivation for behaviour in every sphere. Likewise, performance which is not reinforced by association with peers tends to lag. Families, too, often have stronger and clearer goals for children's achievement once they have reached school age.

Peer influence in the classroom and school playground has been demonstrated notably to have more force in children's language development than does the home environment. In the Sandwell study (Duncan *et al.*, 1985) subjects in those schools with high proportions of Panjabi speaking pupils showed better performance in mother tongue and weaker scores in L2 English on the Sandwell assessment (Duncan *et al.*, 1988) as compared to pupils in those schools with a substantially lower number of Panjabi speakers, while the latter subjects performed better in English as a second language.

Gibbs (1988) showed similar results concerning the L1/L2 ambience in the school environment in a study assessing Panjabi speaking pupils' performance in expressing English modality. Again, subjects in the area of Sandwell where schools have the highest proportion of English mother-tongue pupils had considerably lower mean error scores than those in the two areas with low numbers of English L1 students. A sociolinguistic questionnaire in the same study suggested virtually no effect from home language use influence.

Finally, educational placement practices can exert pressures upon school-aged children. Such difficulties as slow acquisition of oral English or problems with literacy and symbolization can result in children's placement in lower sets and remedial groups within the mainstream school and in the eventual consideration of alternative placement in special provision for them.

The inter-professional team

Who are the professionals who have management responsibilities for the development of the mainstream child exhibiting language deficit? The basic team may be considered to consist of classroom teachers, mother-tongue teachers and second language teachers, plus the speech therapist and educational psychologist. Joint effort on a co-operative basis is of the essence, if all dimensions of the difficulties and welfare of the developing bilingual child are to be accounted for and given their due weight. In addition, ready and effective liaison with the home and other professionals, such as remedial teachers, social workers, community health physicians, medical consultants and audiologists, is essential for insight and information-gathering. This can be accomplished through an interchange of reports, visits and consultations, preferably with the help of bilingual personnel, at every stage of diagnosis and treatment.

THERAPY ISSUES

Group therapy

When assessment is as complete as possible, how then may remediation best be undertaken for bilingual children? There are several considerations which encourage the selection of therapy in small groups rather than individual therapy for this population — the school-aged, mainstream bilingually language handicapped. These reasons are based on therapeutic principles and practical demands.

The basic tenets of **group therapy** are well known — i.e. the group dynamic, linguistic advantages, contra-indications, the practical demands, and so on; however, we will set them out here because it is important that all members of the inter-professional team are familiar with them. Furthermore, if members of the team have not had experience of language work with small groups, then it becomes clear that they must have some training in the group therapy process. The following discussion should be read in the light of delivering therapy in both languages.

Peer models

It has been well documented in the literature that in teacher–peer language-learning situations, children seem to acquire their language from their peers rather than from the teacher. Dulay, Burt and Krashen (1982, p. 30) note 'when both a teacher and peers speak the target language, learners have been observed to prefer the latter as models for themselves'. They cite Milon (1975), Bruck, Lambert and Tucker (1975) and Plann (1977) to this effect. Furthermore, Chesterfield and Chesterfield (1985) have shown that children seem to acquire language in peer-oriented environments rather than through teacher-fronted situations.

Group dynamic

One of the most important opportunities offered by groupwork is that of generating and harnessing the group dynamic. In the classic individual client–therapist situation it is impossible to create anything other than a contrived spontaneity for turn-taking and role-playing. Yet in groupwork these are natural procedures (Travis, 1971).

Having created the group dynamic, the important point to note about harnessing it is that the therapist must know when and how to hand over the dynamic to the group. The result of this will be peer-controlled interaction rather than therapist-controlled interaction. One of the primary challenges for group therapy is introducing activities which are capable of sustaining authentic peer interaction, as well as focusing on and developing the grammatical and pragmatic aims of therapy (Hutt, 1979).

Linguistic aspects

At a time when a more balanced harmony between the various aspects of linguistic development is being sought, group remediation offers more potential for marrying grammatical and pragmatic aims.

Apart from a more natural and authentic environment for language games, groups encourage social skills and social communication because of group members' interaction.

Contra-indications

It has been noted that different groups of children, particularly the language handicapped, will respond in different ways to groupwork. It is the therapist's first challenge to find out how the group of children will work together, and this must be an initial aim in the remediation programme. It can happen that some children do not benefit from groupwork, usually because of the nature and complexity of their disorder. For example, there may be concomitant behaviour problems, or their problems may be of differing severity from those of the candidates being considered for group remediation.

Further, the speech therapist must avoid the temptation of running the group as a conglomerate of 1:1 relationships. She must be prepared to relinquish that special relationship with each child in favour of the group dynamic.

Generalization

The group should resolve the challenge for the child of generating the grammatical structure of therapy to the wider communication context. The problem that 'she can do it in clinic but won't do it outside' should be greatly eased.

Finally, the group situation offers an ongoing display for informal observation which should reflect more accurately the child's everyday peer communication demands than the context of a 1:1 relationship with the therapist. Indications about spontaneous language use and patterns of language use will be obtained. Thus assessment and re-assessment should be more embracing, more appropriate and more accurate in the profile they give of the child's language skills.

Practical demands

There are several practical demands, such as bilingual personnel, timetabling, venue, transport and resources, which evolve from the decision to offer therapy in small groups. They could be seen as disadvantages and as mitigating against groupwork. On the other hand, prior planning can consolidate support for such a project and ensure optimal execution.

Personnel

Two criteria must be met if bilingual group remediation is to be successful. The first is that bilingual input must be available, either a bilingual speech therapist manages the group where she shares the two main languages of the children in the group or a bilingual co-worker provides the mother-tongue input which a monolingual speech therapist does not have at her command. The therapist and co-worker, then, must work closely together to implement the bilingual therapy.

The second criterion is that the group of children must share the same languages — i.e. mother tongue and second language. It is possible to run language-learning groups which are polyglot, but this often means that only the Direct Method of language teaching can be used. That is, there can be little or no teaching of the second language through the mother tongue.

Much more important, this would present enormous problems in the mother-tongue therapy sessions if the co-worker or bilingual therapist had to use two or more languages, even supposing she had fluent command of them, to a polyglot group of language handicapped children in order to render mother-tongue language remediation — e.g. in Panjabi and Gujerati, or Turkish and Greek, or Italian and Spanish. It is possible to argue that such a situation with children of normal language-learning abilities might be successful. However, it would be bound to cause considerable confusion and thus would be therapeutically unacceptable with children who, because of their language-acquisition problems, might well have auditory inhibition problems as well.

Timetable

It would be necessary to organize co-ordinated timetabled sessions for the personnel not only for the remediation, but also for therapy preparation and liaison work. If intensive therapy were selected, and it often is where group therapy is concerned, then perhaps up to one-half of the therapist's and the co-worker's timetable might be dedicated to this type of project.

Attendance and transport

With such consumption of professional time, client attendance becomes a priority, which brings to the forefront the issue of poor attendance and how it can be tackled.

In the case where the same 6–12 clients are expected to be at the same group therapy session two or more times a week for most of the year, then it is practical to organize transport facilities for those clients. This is less complicated if the clients live in a small geographical area, and more difficult if their homes are wide-spread.

The causes which underlie poor attendance at speech therapy clinics are various; and many, such as illness, unpunctuality, double-booking and the emergency, are common to all the sub-cultures in the cosmopolitan community. However, in some subcultures, particularly at the lowest socioeconomic levels, which comprise many of the bilingual, as well as Afro-Caribbean and white populations, then the Establishment — encompassing the health and educational systems — can be associated with unpleasant experiences such as powerlessness. Literacy and appointment cards are associated with demands and summonses, for example, bills and fines. Furthermore, it is known that the public understanding of speech therapy and speech and language handicap is fairly minimal (Enderby and Phillip, 1986). Finally, in many Asian households decisions and actions are only undertaken with permission of the head of the household, not necessarily the parent of the child concerned. For all these reasons, the traditional (white, middle-class) means of approaching clients and their parents (e.g. an appointment card addressed to the parents) might be totally ineffective, with no response to indicate the reason for its ineffectiveness. Organizing group therapy and transport will necessarily involve dealings with the school, home and family, which will certainly clarify the position about client attendance and often ensure attendance.

Venue/resources

Because of the numbers of children involved in groupwork (up to six in any group), therapy accommodation is often challenged. Often teaching material resources are also exposed as being woefully inadequate to cope with group therapy for the bilingually language handicapped. Multicultural materials are needed because they are more sensitive. Materials also need to be specific to the therapy aim. It is often the case that traditional suppliers of therapy materials may not be able to satisfy the requirements of the bilingual therapy programme and local alternatives may have to be explored.

Efficiency

Finally, now that speech therapy has reached an age when it can and must monitor its achievements, good organization can obtain maximum benefits from scarce and expensive resources, for example, transport, bilingual personnel and multicultural materials.

Most important, it can achieve a through-put of bilingually language handicapped children, whereas with 1:1 monolingual therapy little through-put has been registered for the moderate and severe cases. Further, the experience of bilingual group remediation and teamwork are important therapy experiences which add another positive dimension to working and achieving with the language handicapped.

BILINGUAL LANGUAGE THERAPY

The issue about which language should be used in therapy for the bilingually language handicapped child is controversial. Chapter 2 attempted to draw a theoretical framework about bilingual language development for the practitioner as a rationale for making decisions about therapy. Here the salient features which must be borne in mind are the acquisitional as opposed to the learned nature of language growth, the social contexts which language needs for its development and language processes which are similar for both first and second language development, as well as delayed and possibly deviant language growth.

Carrow-Woolfolk and Lynch recommend that:

The severely language-disordered child should be taught one language only and the language of the home and the school should be the same whenever possible. For children with moderate language disorder a single language should be used for instruction, but the language of the home may differ. (Carrow-Woolfolk and Lynch, 1982, pp. 441, 442)

This approach seems to be based on the following assumptions:

1. That language disorder ameliorates more efficiently when language input is restricted and monolingual;
2. That language functions in a social and cultural vacuum;
3. That potentially bilingual children do not need to function in bilingual communities — i.e. that bilingual communities can operate as monolingual communities.

We would strongly argue against these assumptions on empirical and ethical grounds; ethically, the decision on which language would be remediated, with all its social, emotional, cultural and educational implications, would pose a grave responsibility. Halliday (1975, p. 5) points out that: 'a child, in the act of learning language is also learning the culture through language. The semantic system which he is constructing becomes the primary mode of transmission of the culture.' By ignoring or failing to accommodate the mother tongue, one is failing to take on board all the evidence of social and emotional factors which have been shown to be fundamental in language learning — not only in L1, but also in L2 (Okamura-Bichard, 1985). To choose the L2 in preference to the young language handicapped child's mother tongue is to ignore six years of language development and to approach language remediation in a social vacuum. Most 'motherese' studies have shown that one of the most important predisposing factors in language acquisition is a positive social and emotional environment. Bruck (1984), in discussing diagnosis and treatment considerations for children from the minority background with specific learning disabilities in general, and with language disability in particular, notes that 'in addition to psychological and pedagogical factors, one must also consider the sociolinguistic and cultural background of the child and attempt to place him or her in a situation where the mother tongue will not be replaced by the second language, and where pride in his own culture can be fostered' (p. 125).

There is a growing amount of empirical data which supports the notion that offering a bilingually language-disordered system input in both languages promotes language learning in both languages. It could be that the disordered system needs more opportunities, quantitatively and qualitatively, to acquire language patterns. D'Anglejan and Renaud (1985, p. 13) demonstrated in their study that in subjects with classroom anxiety and learning difficulties, 'these were exacerbated by use of low-redundancy structurally based methods allowing little place for hypothesis testing and other processes thought to underlie unconscious second language learning'. Furthermore, Bruck's studies (1978, 1982, 1984) of language disabled Anglophone children attending immersion programmes in L2 French show that the children in the French programme acquired oral proficiency in their mother tongue at the same rate as language-disabled children schooled in English. They also acquired oral proficiency in French, though obviously not at the same rate as their non-handicapped peers. Thus, Bruck (1984, p. 126) points out: 'exposure to and instruction in a weaker language did not confuse these children nor impede their linguistic growth'. By contrast, language-disabled children in the English stream who followed a traditional French L2 programme for 30 minutes a day over a period of three years had acquired no L2 skills. On a smaller scale, Perozzi (1985) looked at how three Spanish speaking pre-schoolers, two of whom were language handicapped, and three English-speaking pre-schoolers could acquire receptive vocabulary in L2 when taught through L1. He found that L2 English receptive vocabulary was learnt significantly faster when the same vocabulary was taught first in the L1. He felt this supported the idea that remediation which started in the L1 would facilitate the remediation of L2.

Finally, Skinner (1985) argues against the use of the Direct

Method approach to L2 instruction. His arguments deal with instruction of normal L2 students, but they equally apply to the remediation of the language handicapped. Briefly, his arguments state, first, that the Direct Method is not appropriate, and secondly, that we should look for methods which link thoughts to words. The Direct Method presumes: (a) that there is language equivalency in an acquisitional manner between L1 English and L2 English, and (b) that the instruction must be done in the L2. One of the points which we shall make in the model for remediation, described below, is an application of an alternative approach to that of the Direct Method with bilingually language handicapped children.

THE SANDWELL PROJECT

Many of the considerations discussed in the preceding pages were taken into account in the establishment of a programme of bilingual group therapy for Panjabi speaking language handicapped children in the Metropolitan Borough of Sandwell, which adjoins Birmingham in the West Midlands. The remediation phase of the project, which was a joint education and health department venture by Sandwell's Ethnic Minorities Support and Speech Therapy services, began in January 1985. The first two and a half years of the remediation programme are presented here; the personnel involved have changed, but these have always involved a speech therapist and two ESL teachers — one of whom is bilingual — with additional training in language development and assessment. From the establishment of the project, the special-needs liaison worker from the Ethnic Minorities Support Service of the education authority has maintained the co-ordination and guidance of the programme.

Model for remediation

The development of the model for remediation was influenced by several practical constraints, as well as two central issues. There was limited access to personnel, treatment rooms, finance and time, but some decisions were made irrespective of these constraints. It is possible, given different resources, that a full-time language unit for more children could have been established, but

187

this would have entailed removing the bilingually language handicapped children from their neighbourhood setting and friends in their local schools, as well as from sound peer models of spoken L1 Panjabi and L1 English for their language development. This provision would have gone against the fundamental philosophy of keeping children with special needs integrated into mainstream education, as adopted in the *Education Act 1981*. Optimally, bilingual treatment would take place on three or four mornings a week, with a further session for planning, recording and materials' development, but this was not possible initially because of constraints on personnel. Thus the decision was taken to offer remediation in L1 Panjabi and L2 English for two mornings a week in a health centre to not more than ten children, aged 6–9 years, found to have depressed profiles in both languages on the diagnostic version of the Sandwell Bilingual Assessment (Duncan *et al.*, 1988).

Selection of pupils

During its first 18 months the project was piloted in Smethwick, one area of the Metropolitan Borough of Sandwell, and pupils were selected from primary schools in that district. Subsequently, education authority taxis were provided, thus making it possible to select children from schools in all parts of the borough.

Referrals for the groups are made, in the first instance, by community therapists and headteachers. The Sandwell Bilingual Assessment of Expressive Panjabi and English and the revised bilingual version of the Wheldall Sentence Comprehension Test (1987) are then administered to the referred children. Pupils with total and subtotal error scores of −2 or −3 standard deviations from the means of their peers in both languages on the expressive language assessment are selected. (Some of the pupils have had mild associated receptive difficulties as well, which generally have ameliorated to within normal limits after a few months of therapy.) The pupils are divided into two language groups with a maximum of five members each on the basis of the similarity of their expressive language profiles and taking into account, in addition, their general level of maturity.

Objectives

The remediation project seeks to establish: (a) that concurrent bilingual structured remediation would have a positive and measurable effect on the grammatical profiles; (b) that ongoing assessment of language structures and language use yields helpful diagnostic information and (c) that confidence, desire and ability to communicate, social language and social dynamic improve.

Therapy

The therapy aims are based on the pupils' linguistic strengths and weaknesses. The Sandwell Bilingual Assessment produces grammatical profiles in both Panjabi and English, and observation yields information about semantic and communicative abilities. Therapy intends to build up the profiles into a more balanced normal pattern. Developmental sequence of language acquisition does not dictate remediation for two reasons. First, it is not yet available in L1 Panjabi; and secondly, some of the profiles in L2 English have not reflected developmental delay, but more deviant acquisition, so that developmental information is used as a guideline only where appropriate.

The desirability of structured input for remediation with English language-disabled children is well established. Hutt (1986, p. 5) has reflected on the early attempts of the John Horniman School to form a curriculum: 'It gradually became apparent that both the content of the curriculum and the methods of presenting it must be highly structured.'.

Remediation aims are always first introduced into therapy receptively, before children are expected to express a structure, that is the children are given ample opportunity to develop semantic and pragmatic awareness of the syntactic structure, as well as being offered a good sound model. The children are encouraged to use grammatical structures functionally, in appropriate contexts. For example, a child could be requested to go to the teacher of the other group and ask her or him: 'Can I have my book, please?'.

The morning is timetabled in two halves, to allow the two groups of children to have remediation in both languages. The sessions are structured, commencing with social greetings, moving into the receptive task of the objective, then to the expressive task. Most activities involve turn-taking, which provide a satisfactory way of closing. Both the receptive and expressive work have been extended where appropriate to visual work. It is often necessary for vocabulary work to precede the introduction of structures. The

189

main thrust of the actitivies is to encourage and establish group dynamic and inter-child communication. To this end, dialogue and role-play are employed, initiating the task to peers and 'acting out' a scenario for verbs, tense change and interrogatives. No drills are used, and responses in unison are sometimes employed, as in pantomimic usage — 'Oh, yes he is!' A mid-morning break further encourages social interaction, when the children usually opt to speak L1 Panjabi. Bilingual teaching is sometimes used by the Panjabi speaking teacher to help the children in the more advanced group (aged 7½ plus) develop English L2 structures for which the parallel Panjabi syntax is already well established. Relating of past events and retelling stories in both languages, to help establish irregular and regular past tense structures in L2 English, are activities where this strategy is particularly beneficial. The children's acquisition of English structures is found to be more sound with the use of both languages than when English syntax is taught only through English.

Materials

Often browsing through shops in the local area has provided appropriate visuals. Commercial visual materials are frequently found to be inappropriate, particularly regarding lexis, not least because each commercial pack tends to select a different set of lexical items for the same structures.

   Teaching literacy of reinforce oral language work has been monitored; it has been beneficial for some children, who seem better able to retain the structures orally after experiencing their written form. However, a number of children find the array of words in the pupils' folders confusing and only the teacher's large word cards are helpful; others do not seem able to benefit from written language input for some time. A modified set of word cards for Panjabi has been developed, using English orthography. However, its use is equivocal for several reasons. First, the use of this orthography has no carry-over value for reading and writing in any other setting. It has not been possible to teach the childen Gurmukhi script, even if that had been desirable, because that script is used only by the Sikh community, whereas the Sikh and Muslim communities have always been coincidentally represented about equally in the groups of children. Secondly, only a slight proportion of remediation time can be allotted to literacy work in the first place, and consequently it has not seemed practical to introduce reading and writing in more than one language. The whole area of materials for ethnolinguistic remediation would bear further research and development.

Planning the remediation

Planning is conducted as follows:

1. Termly, following assessment/reassessment, to set aims for remediation;
2. Half-termly, to amend termly aims in the light of progress;
3. Weekly, to develop or amend objectives to the aims and to plan lesson activities.

Discussion always follows the assessment of a child, and ideas about remediation aims are suggested. Planning is usually done separately for Panjabi L1 and English L2, and aims for the two languages are not usually the same. This approach is dictated by preference and need. Remediation, in parallel, on similar syntactic structures in L1 and L2 might cause confusion. Furthermore, the need to remediate similiar structures in L1 and L2 does not normally present itself in the assessment profiles of the children. So, for example, during one particular term L1 Panjabi worked on past and future verb tenses, while L2 English remediation included copula and auxiliary structures and interrogatives.

Recording and liaison

After each session, a brief résumé is made of each child's responses — successful or otherwise — to the session's objectives. Sometimes it also includes other pertinent information, for example, behaviour and health. Copies of these résumés are sent back to the schools weekly, and termly progress reports are written, with copies sent to the schools and to officers of other agencies involved with the children such as the educational psychologist, audiologist, ENT consultant and community medical officers. Liaison is supplemented by termly visits to the schools by the speech therapist, as well as meetings of the ESL teachers who do English language work with the members of the groups in their schools. Where there are mother-tongue teachers, they too could be involved. The Panjabi teacher visits the children's homes at least once a term, in order that parents can reinforce the Panjabi therapy. The two ESL teachers involved in the project have monitored the progress in the classroom, both of those children currently in the groups and those who have been discharged. This practice has aimed to ensure that the progress which has been shown in the clinic remediation sessions is incorporated into classroom work, both on a short- and long-term basis. There is also frequent and ongoing liaison with the educational psychologists in the areas of the children's schools and with the relevant health visitors and community health physicians.

Table 11.1 Total error scores for language-handicapped pupils

	1		2		3	
	(L1)	*(L2)*	*(L1)*	*(L2)*	*(L1)*	*(L2)*
Subject:						
A1	47*	U	42	96	41	82
	—	—	−3SD	−3SD	−3SD	−3SD
A2	22	64	27	76	17	67
	−1SD	−3SD	−1SD	−3SD	−1SD	−3SD
B	40†	U	40*	59*	26	65
	—	—	—	—	−2SD	−2SD
C	26*	74	29	69	14	51
	—	−3SD	−1SD	−2SD	+1SD	−1SD
D	U	49*	49*	50	NA	39
	—	—	—	−1SD	—	−1SD
E	U	70	22	67	5	56
	—	−2SD	−1SD	−2SD	+1SD	−3SD
F	U	68	37	59	18	26
	—	−2SD	−2SD	−2SD	+1SD	+1SD
G	U	U	39	73	24	39
	—	—	−2SD	−3SD	−1SD	−1SD
H	U	76	39	73	23	52
	—	−3SD	−2SD	−3SD	−1SD	−2SD
I	47	U	—	73	14	58
	−3SD	—	—	−3SD	−1SD	−3SD
J	22	64	27	76	17	67
	−1SD	−3SD	−1SD	−3SD	−1SD	−3SD
K	46*	67	33	57	16	45
	—	−2SD	−2SD	−3SD	−1SD	−3SD
L	30	69	22	66	13	53
	−2SD	−2SD	−1SD	−2SD	+1SD	−3SD

Key: U = unassessable
* = interrogative section not administered
† = testing abandoned
SD = standard deviation(s).

Results

The results discussed here are based on the assessment/re-assessment scores of 14 out of the 20 or so children who have attended this programme over two and a half years. The children's grammatical development has been quantified into raw scores obtained from the total scores for their performance on the Sandwell Bilingual Assessment of Panjabi and English, measured three times at six-monthly intervals (Table 11.1). The raw data are incompatible with statistical analysis, but they have been used to draw up tables of quantitative changes in subjects' language behaviour over three of their assessments. They show the number of subjects whose scores have dropped over the three assessments, those whose scores have risen and those whose scores have remained the same. 'Uncomparable data' means that a subject did not perform for a particular category or for a whole assessment. Pupil A, who has attended for the entire period that the programme has run, with the exception of a term's absence for a visit to India, has data for six assessments instead of the usual three.

Discussion

The first objective is to establish whether concurrent bilingual structured remediation has a positive and measurable effect on the grammatical profiles. The data suggests that this aim has been fulfilled. The total error scores of all of the subjects went down in both languages (Table 11.1). These children have a genuine language-acquisition problem. The assessment results of children who presented with depressed language profiles for other reasons, for example, social or emotional, are not included in the data; however, initial assessments for two of these children appear in Table 11.2.

It could be argued that the measured improvement is in line with that due to the passage of time, rather than remediation, since no control group was involved. This criticism stands because there is no statistical analysis of the data, and no control group for comparison. Anecdotally, it can be said that data exists for children on speech therapy waiting-lists who have been assessed and re-assessed, showing very little improvement over 12 months without therapy. Also from clinical experience the authors can say that there has been improvement in the English of bilingually language handicapped children after intensive L2 English intervention, although the mother-tongue Panjabi had improved only slightly or not at all.

The important finding is that these data show that concurrent bilingual remediation does not have a negative effect on the language of bilingually language handicapped children. It would seem to contradict the line of approach put forward by Carrow-Woolfolk and Lynch (1982) and others, and to support the idea that offering more linguistic stimuli — qualitatively and quanti-tatively — has a beneficial effect on the bilingual language development of bilingually handicapped children.

At this stage, it is not possible to define which aspect of remedi-ation has been responsible for the linguistic improvement — i.e. the structured input, the use of strategies and the group dynamic. Most probably, all the aspects together have constituted an envi-ronment which has encouraged language development.

It is important to note that if a monolingual approach to the treatment of these bilingual language handicapped children were the right one, and had input in two languages concurrently been strongly contra-indicated, definite disimprovements would have been measured in the total error scores. Could it be said that perhaps the language improvement was slowed down by being done bilingually? More data needs to be gathered to compare L2 English only intervention with L1/L2 intervention. Even if there were a significant or even sizeable difference in favour of the L2 English only intervention, would it be justified in terms of all the linguistic needs of the bilingual child? It is worth noting that three of the subjects had expressive Panjabi performances within normal limits at their third assessment. In addition to overall language development, measurable improvement took place for most of the pupils on the structures introduced in the remediation during the term in which they were taught.

The second objective is to discover whether ongoing assessment of language structures and language use yields helpful diagnostic information. Ongoing assessment has been able to differentiate lines of action for three categories of children: those for whom language difficulties are primary; those whose similar grammatical profiles are depressed due to social or emotional/behavioural problems; and those with learning/perceptual problems. Struc-tured language input often results in rapid progress for pupils in the second category, so that quite soon their profiles reflect

Table 11.2 Total error scores for two pupils

| | 1 | | 2 | |
	(L1)	(L2)	(L1)	(L2)
Subject:				
A	U	U	21	67
			M	−3SD
B	U	U	18	69
			+1SD	−3SD

Key: U = unassessable
M = score at the mean for peer group
SD = standard deviation(s).

language behaviour within the normal limits for their peer group, as with the L1 data in Table 11.2. Thus these children are fairly quickly discernible from those with genuine language-learning disability.

The two pupils in the table, having already demonstrated mother-tongue expression at or above the mean for their peers after only two terms of remediation, were discharged after one further term's work to reinforce the establishment of their L2 structures. So, too, Kalvinder and Ravinder, both girls whose home circumstances were disrupted and whose behaviour was disturbed, were placed on review with improved expression after two terms in the group (data not included). There is another group of children who fail to respond because the remediation is not designed to help with their primary problems. Jagdeep and Abdul were discharged after two terms because they were found to have global learning disabilities and were unable to benefit from the remediation. Zahid was discharged when his oral expression in both languages was assessed as within normal limits for his peer group after four terms' bilingual help and he was referred for assessment and remediation in literacy skills.

Of those pupils clearly manifesting language handicap, a number of subsidiary problems have been diagnosed. One pupil, Ahmed, whose eyesight was 6/9 when he joined the group, became increasingly unable to respond to visual stimuli during the sessions. On referral, his sight was found to have deteriorated within one year to 6/60, possibly as a manifestation of a genetic disorder. The same pupil presents with ENT problems, including dysphonia and mild hearing loss. One boy, Sarbjit, was fitted with a hearing aid with a high-frequency loop. In addition, after nearly two years of bilingual remediation, he had finally acquired sufficient expressive ability in both languages that his misordered phonology and receptive disability were manifest. At that point, he was placed in a full-time unit. Another boy, Abid, was found to have unilateral nerve deafness, and yet another boy and a girl were diagnosed as having moderate conductive loss, requiring minor surgery. Thus termly medical examinations are crucial, and the team facilitates liaison between parents, schools and medical officers with regard to appointments and further referrals.

The third objective is to establish that confidence and motivation to communicate, as well as social language, will improve. That aim is the most difficult to assess because it relies on subjective reports and implicit data, yet it yields the most obvious results. There are three indicators of improvement. First, all the subjects have improved in their confidence and desire to talk both to each other and to adults in the clinic setting. This has been substantiated by observations of termly visitors to the remediation project. Secondly, improvement in the home and in the school has been indicated by favourable reports from parents and teachers. One boy, Gurdev, who had not spoken to anyone in school for the whole of the previous academic year, began to make friends, speak to teachers and enthusiastically join activities from which he had previously withdrawn completely. Finally, it has been noted by the children's increasing ability to cope with the assessment tools. Eight of the 14 subjects were unable to respond on one scale of the initial language assessment, but they became assessable after six months or more of therapy. The Sandwell project has shown that bilingual group remediation has been notably beneficial for the children who have participated in it.

CONCLUSION

This chapter has discussed the challenges that are encountered when providing therapy for the bilingual language handicapped child. These challenges are best met when there is access to both of the child's languages for assessment and therapy through working with a bilingual team. It is clear that more research must be conducted into developing and using appropriate materials and resources with this client group.

The projects described in this chapter and in Chapter 8 provide models for bilingual therapy but more documentation is needed, both about other ways of delivering therapy and about working with different pathology groups in the bilingual population. Here we have tried to show that it is the same therapeutic principles which underlie therapy whether it be to monolingual or bilingual language handicapped children. We have also tried to indicate how the implementation of these principles has been modified to meet the specific needs of the bilingual population. Although there will always be a place for individual therapy, the group model with bilingual input has enormous potential for language handicapped children.

Bibliography

Abudarham, S. (1980) The role of the speech therapist in the assessment of the language-learning potential and proficiency of children with dual language systems or backgrounds. *Journal of Multilingual and Multicultural Development*, **1** (3), 187–206.

Abudarham, S. (1984) The use of interpreters in the assessment of the languages of children with dual language systems. *Proceedings of Congress of IALP.*

Abudarham, S. (1987) *Bilingualism and the Bilingual: An interdisciplinary approach to pedagogic and remedial issues*, NFER-Nelson, Windsor.

Acosta-Belan, E. (1975) Spanglish: case of languages in contact. In *New Directions in Second Language Learning, Teaching and Bilingual Education*, (eds M. Burt and H. Dulay), Papers of Ninth TESOL Convention, Los Angeles, Calif., USA, pp. 151–8.

Advisory Centre For Education (ACE) (1981) *A Summary of the Education Act*, ACE, London.

Ahmed, S. (1982) Translation is at best an echo. *Community Care*, 22 April, pp. 19–21.

Aitchison, J. (1976) *The Articulate Mammal*, Hutchinson, London.

Alderson, J.C. (1980) Native and non-native speaker performance on cloze tests. *Language Learning*, **30** (1), 54–76.

Andersen, R.W. (1977) The impoverished state of cross-sectional morpheme acquisition accuracy and methodology. *Working Papers in Bilingualism*, **14**, 47–82.

Bailey, P. and Jenkinson, J. (1976) The application of Blissymbolics. *Special Education: Forward Trends*, **3**, September.

Baker, R. and Briggs, J. (1975) Working with interpreters in social work practice. *Australian Social Work*, **28** (4) 31–7.

Ball, M. and Jones, G. (1984) *Welsh Phonology: Selected Readings*, University of Wales Press, Cardiff.

Bardsley, J. and Perkins, E. (1983) Portage with Asian families in Central Birmingham. Paper delivered at Third National Portage Conference, UK.

Barnett, P. (1983) The role of the speech therapist in the diagnosis and remediation of language handicap among the nursery school population within the Newham Health District. Unpublished (available from The Speech Therapy Department, 84 West Ham Lane, London E15 4PT).

Barnett, P. and Fletcher-Wood, V. (1981) *Let's Play Language*. LDA, Wisbech.

Barnett, S. and Stokes, J. (1985) Speech therapy, bilingualism and associated issues: a report on a national survey. *Bulletin*, (College of Speech Therapists), July, pp. 2–3.

Bates, E. (1976) Pragmatics and sociolinguistics in child language. In *Language Deficiency in Children: Selected readings,* (eds D. and A. Morehead).

Beheydt, L. (1984) The semantic primacy principle in motherese. Paper presented at Child Language Seminar, Nottingham University, March.

Bloom, L. (1970) *Language Development: Forms and Functions in Emerging Grammars,* MIT Press, Cambridge, Mass.

Bloom, L. and Lahey, C. (1978) *Language Development and Language Disorders,* Wiley, New York and London.

Brent-Palmer, C. (1979) Sociolinguistic assessment of the notion im/ migrant semilingualism from a social conflict perspective. *Working Papers in Bilingualism,* **17,** 137–80.

Brown, R. (1973) *A First Language: The Early Stages,* Allen and Unwin, London.

Bruck, M. (1978) The suitability of early French immersion programs for the language disabled child. *Canadian Journal of Education,* **3,** 51–72.

Bruck, M. (1982) Language impaired child performance in an additive bilingual education program. *Applied Psycholinguistics,* **3,** (1) 45–60.

Bruck, M. (1984) The suitability of immersion education for children with special needs. In *Communicative Competence Approaches to Language Proficiency Assessment: Research and Application,* (ed. C. Rivera), pp. 123–31. No. 9 in the series Multilingual Matters, Multilingual Matters Ltd., Avon.

Bruck, M., Lambert, W. and Tucker, G. (1975) Assessing functional bilingualism within a bilingual program: the St Lambert project at grade eight. Paper presented at TESOL Convention, Los Angeles, Calif., USA.

Bruner, J. (1975) The ontogenesis of speech acts. *Journal of Child Language,* **2** (1), 1–19.

Campbell, S.J. (1986) Community interpreting and translation in Australia. *Linguist,* **25,** (2) 66–8.

Carrow-Woolfolk, E. and Lynch, J. (1982) *An Integrative Approach to Language Disorders in Children,* Grune and Stratton, New York.

Carter, A. (1984) The acquisition of social deixis — children's usage of kin terms in Maharashra, India. *Journal of Child Language,* **11** (1), 179–201.

Chana, U. and Romaine, S. (1984) Evaluative reactions to Panjabi/ English code-switching. *Journal of Multilingual and Multicultural Development,* **5** (6), 447–73.

Chapman, R. (1981) Computing mean length of utterance in morphemes. In *Assessing Language Production in Children,* (ed. J.E. Miller), Edward Arnold, London.

Chesterfield, R. and Chesterfield, K.B. (1985) Natural order in children's use of second language learning strategies. *Applied Linguistics,* **6** (1), 45–59.

Child, E. (1982) Individual and social factors associated with behaviour of children in a play setting. Unpublished PhD thesis, Aston University, Birmingham, UK.

Chomsky, C.S. (1969). *The Acquisition of Syntax in Children from 5 to*

10, MIT Press, Cambridge, Mass.

Clark, E. (1973) What's in a word? On the child's acquisition of semantics in his first language. In *Cognitive Development and the Acquisition of Language* (ed. T. Moore), Academic Press, New York, pp. 65–110.

Cohen, and Manion, (1985) *Research Methods in Education,* Croom Helm, London.

Commission for Racial Equality (CRE) (1978) *Caring for the Under-fives in a Multiracial Society,* Commission for Racial Equality, London.

Cooper, J. Moodley, M. and Reynell, J, (1978) *Helping Language Development,* Edward Arnold, London.

Corsellis, A. (1984) *Outline of the Tasks of an Interpreter.* (Available from the Speech Therapy and Bilingualism Resource Centre, Department of Continuing Education, Chandler House, 2 Wakefield Street, London WC1N 1PG.)

Corsellis, A. (1986) Interpretation in the courts and the police and probation services. In *Witnesses,* Report by JUSTICE, London.

Corsellis, A. (1988) The Community Interpreter Project. *Linguist,* **27** (1), 16–19.

Crystal, D. (1982) *Profiling Language Disability,* Edward Arnold, London.

Crystal, D. (1987) *Clinical Linguistics,* Edward Arnold, London.

Crystal, D., Garman, M. and Fletcher, P. (1976) *The Grammatical Analysis of Language Disability: A Procedure for Assessment and Remediation,* Edward Arnold, London.

Cummins, J. (1979) Linguistic independence and the educational development of bilingual children. *Review of Education Research,* **49** (2), 222–51.

Cummins, J. (1980) *Psychological Assessment of Minority Language Students* (Final Report), Ontario Institute for Studies in Education.

Damico, J., Oller, J. and Storey, M. (1981) The diagnosis of language disorders in bilingual children: pragmatic and surface-orientated criteria. In *The Bilingual Exceptional Child* (eds. J. Erikson and D. Omark) Charles C. Thomas, Springfield, Ill.

Damico, J., Oller, J. and Storey, M. (1983) The diagnosis of language disorders in bilingual children: surface-orientated and pragmatic criteria. *Journal of Speech and Hearing Disorders,* **48** (4), 385–94.

D'Anglejan, A. and Renaud, C. (1985) Learner characteristics and second language acquisition: a multivariate study of adult immigrants and some thoughts on methodology. *Language Learning,* **35**, 1–19.

Day, R.R. (1979) The acquisition and maintenance of language by minority children. *Language Learning,* **29** (2), 295.

Department of Health and Social Security (DHSS) (1984) *Interdepartmental group on provision for under-fives: services for under-fives from ethnic minority communities.* HMSO, London.

Dore, J. (1975) Holophrases, speech acts and language universals. *Journal of Child Language,* **2**, 21–40.

Dulay, H. and Burt, M. (1974) Natural sequences in child second language acquisition. *Language Learning* **24**, 37–53.

Dulay, H. and Burt, M. (1977) Some remarks on creativity in second language acquisition. In *Viewpoints on English as a Second Language* (eds M. Burt, H. Dulay and M. Finnochiaro), Regent Press, New York, pp. 95–126.

Dulay, H., Burt, M. and Krashen, S. (1982) *Language Two*, Oxford University Press, Oxford.

Duncan, D. & Gibbs, D. (1987) The acquisition of syntax in Panjabi and English. *British Journal of Disorders of Communication*, **22** (2), 129–44.

Duncan, D., Gibbs, D., Noor, N. and Whittaker, H. (1985). Bilingual acquisition of L1 Punjabi and L2 English by Sandwell primary school children. *ITL Review of Applied Linguistics*, **70**, 1–32.

Duncan, D., Gibbs, D., Noor, N. and Whittaker, H. (1988) *Sandwell Bilingual Screening Assessment Scales for Expressive Panjabi and English*, NFER-Nelson, Windsor.

Ellis, R. (1981) The role of input in language acquisition: some implications for second language teaching. *Applied Linguistics*, **2** (1), 70–82.

Ellis, R. (1984) Discussant. In *Interlanguage*, (eds A. Davies, C. Criper and A.P.R. Howatt), Edinburgh University Press, Edinburgh, pp. 280–6.

Enderby, P. and Phillip, R. (1986) Speech and language handicap: towards knowing the size of the problem. *British Journal of Disorders of Communication*, **21** (2), 151–65.

Fathman, A. (1975) The relationship between age and second language productive ability. *Language Learning*, **25** (2), 245–53.

French, S. (1987) Action research: a flexible approach. *Therapy Weekly*, **14** (9), 7.

Gallagher, T.M. and Prutting, C. (eds) (1983) *Pragmatic Assessment and Intervention Issues in Language*, College-Hill Press, San Diego, Calif.

Galloway, P. (1978) Blissymbols in the classroom. *Special Education: Forward Trends*, **5** (2), 19–21.

Gibbs, D. (1988) Second language acquisition of the English modal auxiliaries 'can', 'could', 'may' and 'might' by Panjabi-speaking pupils. Unpublished PhD thesis, Birmingham Polytechnic, Birmingham.

Gill, D. and Bath, K.S. (1976) *English and Panjabi Grammar and Syntax Comparison*. NAME, Buckingham.

Gill, H.S. and Gleason, H. (1962) *A Reference Grammar of Panjabi*. Hartford, Conn.

Grunwell, P. (1982) *Clinical Phonology*, Croom Helm, London.

Halliday, M. (1973) *Explorations in the Functions of Language*, Edward Arnold, London.

Halliday, M. (1975) *Learning How To Mean*, Edward Arnold, London.

Halsey, A.H. (ed.) (1972) *Educational Priority. Volume 1, EPA Problems and Policies*, HMSO, London.

Hammond, J. and Bailey, P. (1976) An experiment in Blissymbolics. *Special Education: Forward Trends*, **3** (3) 21–2.

Harris, M. (1984) Individual differences in the acquisition of number markers. Paper presented at the Child Language Seminar, Nottingham University, March.

Haugen, E. (1977) Norm and deviation in bilingual communities. In *Bi-*

lingualism: Psychological, Social and Educational Implications (ed. P. Hornby), Academic Press, New York, pp. 91–102.

Home Affairs Select Committee (1981) *Reports on Racial Disadvantage.* HMSO, London.

Howe, C.J. (1981) Interpretive analysis and role semantics: A ten year mesalliance. *Journal of Child Language,* 8, 439–56.

Howlin, P. (1984) Parents as Therapists: a critical review. In D. Miller (ed.) *Remediating Children's Language,* Croom Helm, London.

Hutt, E. (1979) John Horniman School. In *Working With LARSP* (ed. D. Crystal), Edward Arnold, London, pp. 153–78.

Hutt, E. (1986) *Teaching Language-Disordered Children: A Structured Curriculum,* Edward Arnold, London.

Inner London Education Authority (ILEA) (1979–87) Language Census, 1979, 1981, 1983, 1985, 1987. (Available from Research and Statistics Department, ILEA, County Hall, London SE1).

Institute of Linguists' Educational Trust (1987) *The Bilingual Skills Certificate: An Approach to Training and Qualification.* (Available from Institute of Linguists, 24a Highbury Grove, London N5 2EA.)

Jackson, H. (1979) Errors of Punjabi learners of English: a comparison of the grammars of Punjabi and English. *Core 3/3.* Also: (1980) *ITL Review of Applied Linguistics* 55, 69–91.

Jackson, H. (1987) Grammatical features of North Indian languages. In *Bilingualism and the Bilingual* (ed. S. Abudarham), NFER-Nelson, Windsor, pp. 66–74.

James, A.G. (1974) *Sikh Children in Britain,* Oxford University Press, Oxford.

Johnston, J.R. and Slobin, D.I. (1979) The development of locative expressions in English, Italian, Serbo-Croatian and Turkish. *Journal of Child Language* 6, 529–45.

Kessler, C. (1984) Language acquisition in bilingual children. In *Bilingualism and Language Disability,* (ed. N. Miller) Croom Helm, London, pp. 26–54.

Krashen, S. (1978) Is the 'natural order' an artefact of the BSM? *Language Learning,* 28 (1), 187–91.

Krashens, S. (1981) *Second Language Acquisition and Second Language Learning,* Pergamon, Oxford.

Krashen, S. (1982) *Schooling and Language Minority Students: A Theoretical Framework,* Evaluation, Dissemination and Assessment Center. California State University, Los Angeles, Calif.

Krashen, S., Long, M. and Scarcella, R. (1979) Age, rate and eventual attainment in second language acquisition. *TESOL Quarterly,* 13 (4), 573–82.

Labov, W. (1972) *Sociolinguistic Patterns,* University of Pennsylvania Press, Philadelphia, Pa.

Labov, W. (1972) The logic of non-standard English. In *Language and Social Context* (ed. P.P. Gigliodi), Penguin, Harmondsworth.

Lado, R. (1957) *Linguistics across Cultures,* University of Michigan Press, Ann Arbor, Mich.

Leonard, L.B., Steckol, K.F. and Panther, K.M. (1983) Returning meaning to semantic relations: some clinical applications. *Journal of Speech and Hearing Disorders,* **48**, 25–36.

Leopold, W.F. (1970) *Speech Development of a Bilingual Child: A Linguist's Record,* Vols. 1–4; reprinted AMS Press, New York.

Lieven, E. (1984) Interaction style and children's language learning. Paper delivered at the Child Language Seminar, Nottingham University, March.

Lightbown, P. (1984) In *Interlanguage,* (eds A. Davies, C. Criper and A.R.P. Howatt), Edinburgh University Press, Edinburgh, pp. 241–52.

Linguistic Minorities Project (LMP) (1985) *The Other Languages of England* (ed. Michael Stubbs), Routledge and Kegan Paul, London.

London Borough of Newham (1984) *Newham Digest of Census Statistics Second Supplement: Newham's Ethnic Minorities Communities.*

London Interpreting Project (LIP) (1985) *'Training', 'Funding': Some Issues to be Considered in Relation to the Need for Interpreting Services.* (Available from LIP, 245a Coldharbour Lane, London SW9 8RR.)

Long, M.H. and Porter, P.A. (1985) Group work, interlanguage talk and second language acquisition. *TESOL Quarterly,* **19** (2), 207–28.

Lowe, M. (1975) Trends in the development of representational play: an observation study. *Journal of Child Psychology and Psychiatry,* **16**, 33–47.

Lund, N. and Duchan, J. (1983) *Assessing Children's Language in Naturalistic Contexts,* Prentice-Hall, Englewood Cliffs, NJ.

McConkey, R. (1984) The assessment of representational play. In *Remediating Children's Language* (ed. D. Müller), Croom Helm, London.

McCune-Nicholich, L. (1981) Towards symbolic functioning: structure of early pretend games and potential parallels with play. *Child Development,* **52**, 785–97.

McDonald, E.T. (1982) *Teaching and Using Blissymbolics.* Garden City Press, New York.

McGown, M.P. (1982) Guidance for parents of a handicapped child. *Child: Care, Health and Development,* **8** (5), 295–303.

McLaughlin, B. (1978) *Second Language Acquisition in Childhood,* Lawrence Erlbaum, Hillsdale, NJ.

McLean, J. and Synder-McLean, L. (1984) Recent developments in pragmatics: remedial implications. In *Remediating Children's Language* (ed. N. Muller), Croom Helm, London.

McTear, M. (1985) *Children's Conversation,* Basil Blackwell, Oxford.

Mahoney, G.J. and Seeley, P.B. (1976) The role of the social agent in language acquisition: implications for language intervention. In *International Review of Research in Mental Retardation* (ed. N.R. Ellis), Academic Press, New York.

Malik, F. (1987) Getting on speaking terms. *Openmind,* February, p. 5.

Martin-Jones, M. and Romaine, S. (1986). Semilingualism: a half-baked theory of communicative competence. *Applied Linguistics,* **7** (1), 26–38.

Mattes, L. and Omark, D. (1984) *Speech and Language Assessment for the Bilingual Language Handicapped,* College-Hill Press, San Diego, Calif.

Mazurkewich, I. (1983) Syntactic markedness and language acquisition.

Paper presented at Seventh Annual TESOL Convention, Toronto.

Meara, P. (1984) The study of lexis in interlanguage. In *Interlanguage* (eds A. Davies, C. Criper and A.R.P. Howatt), Edinburgh University Press, Edinburgh, pp. 225–36.

Mercer, J. (1973) *Labelling the Mentally Retarded.* University of California Press, Berkeley, Calif.

Miller, J. (1981) *Assessing Language Production In Children,* Edward Arnold, London.

Miller, N. (1979) The bilingual child in the speech therapy clinic. *British Journal of Disorders of Communication,* **13** (1), 17–30.

Miller, N. (ed.) (1984) *Bilingualism and Language Disability — Assessment and Remediation,* Croom Helm, London/College-Hill Press, San Diego, Calif.

Milon, J. (1975) Dialect in the TESOL program: if you never better. In *New Directions in Second Language Teaching and Bilingual Education,* (eds M. Burt and H. Dulay), TESOL, Washington, DC, pp. 159–67.

Mobbs, M. (1982) *Britain's South Asian Languages,* Centre for Information on Language Teaching, London.

Moffatt, S. (1985) Lessons from India. *Bulletin* (College Of Speech Therapists), December, pp. 1–2.

Multi-Ethnic Women's Health Project (1985) *Health Advocacy for Non-English-Speaking Women.* (Available from MEWHP, City and Hackney Community Health Council, 210 Kingsland Road, London E2 8EB.

Munro, S. (1985) An empirical study of specific communication disorders in bilingual children. Unpublished PhD thesis, University of Wales, Cardiff.

Newport, E.L., Gleitman, H. and Gleitman, L.R. (1977) 'Mother, I'd rather do it myself': some effects and non-effects of maternal speech style. In *Talking to Children: Language Input and Acquisition* (eds C.E. Snow and C.A. Ferguson), Cambridge University Press, Cambridge.

Nwokah, E. (1984) Simultaneous and sequential language acquisition in Nigerian children. *First Language,* **5,** 57–73.

Office of Population Censuses and Surveys (OPCS) Monitor Labour Force Survey (1985) *Ethnic Group and Country of Birth.* Government and Statistical Service, ref. LFS 86/2 and PP1 86/3.

Okamura-Bichard, F. (1985) Mother-tongue maintenance and second language learning: a case of Japanese children. *Language Learning,* **35** (1), 63–9.

Omark, D. and Erikson, J. (1983) *The Bilingual Exceptional Child.* College-Hill Press, San Diego, Calif.

Perozzi, J. (1985) A pilot study of language facilitation for bilingual language-handicapped children: theoretical and intervention implications. *Journal of Speech and Hearing Disorders,* **50,** 403–6.

Plann, S. (1977) Acquiring a second language in an immersion classroom. *Teaching and Learning English as a Second Language: Trends in Research and Practice* (eds H.B. Brown, C.A. Yorio and R. Crymes),

TESOL, Washington, DC, pp. 213–25.

Porch, B. (1974) *The Porch Index of Communicative Ability for Children (PICAC)*. Consulting Psychologist Press, Palo Alto, Calif.

Powell, M. and Perkins, E. (1984) Asian families with a pre-school handicapped child; a study. *Mental Handicap,* **12** (2), 50–1.

Prutting, C. (1982) Pragmatics as social competence. *Journal of Speech and Hearing Disorders,* **47** (2), 123–34.

Quirk, R. (1972) *Speech Therapy Services.* HMSO, London.

Quirk, R., Greenbaum, S., Leech, G. and Svartvik, J. (1985) *A Comprehensive Grammar of the English Language,* Longman, New York.

Randell, J. (1985) Negative evidence from positive. Paper presented at Child Language Seminar, Reading University, 1985.

Redlinger, W. and Park, T.-Z. (1980) Language mixing in young bilinguals. *Journal of Child Language,* **7** (2) 337.

Rees, O.A. and Fitzgerald, F. (1981) The Mother-Tongue and English-English Teaching Project. Unpublished report, Department of Education and Science, London.

Rescorla, L. and Okuda, S. (1984) The lexical development in second language acquisition: initial stages in a Japanese child's learning of English. *Journal of Child Language,* **11** (3), 689–95.

Reynell, J. (1986) *The Reynell Developmental Language Scales (RDLS) (Revised),* NFER-Nelson, Windsor.

Rosch, E. (1973) On the internal structure of perceptual and semantic categories. In *Cognitive Development and the Acquisition of Language* (ed. T. Moore), Academic Press, New York.

Shackman, J. (1983) *The Right to be Understood,* National Extension College, London.

Skinner, D. (1985) Access to meaning: the anatomy of the language learning connection. *Journal of Multilingual and Multicultural Development,* **6** (5), 369–88.

Skutnabb-Kangas, T. (1978) Semilingualism and the education of migrant children as a means of reproducing the caste of assembly line workers. In *Papers from the First Scandinavian German Symposium on the Language of Immigrant Workers and their Children* (eds N. Dittmar and U. Teleman), Roskilde: Roskilde Universitet Center, Linguistgruppen, March.

Skutnabb-Kangas, T. (1981) Tvasprakighet Lund: Liber Laromedel.

Skutnabb-Kangas, T. (1984) *Bilingualism or Not: The Education of Minorities,* Multilingual Matters, Avon.

Skutnabb-Kangas, T. and Toukomaa, P. (1976) *Teaching Migrant Children's Mother-Tongue and Learning the Language of the Host Country in the Context of the Socio-cultural Situation of the Migrant Family. Report Prepared for Unesco,* Research Report, No. 15, Department of Sociology and Social Psychology, University of Tampere, Tampere, Finland.

Slobin, D. (1970) Universals of grammatical development in children. In *Advances in Psycholinguistics* (eds G.B. Flores D'Arcais and W.T.M. Levelt), Elsevier, Amsterdam.

Smith, G. (1982) *The Geography and Demography of South Asian*

Languages in England: Some Methodological Problems, Linguistic Minorities Project Working Paper No. 2, Community Languages and Education Project, Institute of Education, University of London.

Smith, G. (1985) *Language, Ethnicity, Employment*, Education and *Research: The Struggle of Sylheti-speaking People in London*, Community Languages and Education Project, Institute of Education, University of London.

Snow, C. (1978) The conversational context of language learning. In *Recent Advances in the Psychology of Language: Language Development and Mother–Child Interaction* (eds R.N. Campbell and P. Smith), Plenum Press, New York.

Spradlin, J.E. and Siegel, G.M. (1982) Language training in natural and clinical environment. *Journal of Speech and Hearing Disorders*, **47** (1), 2–6.

Tolstaya, N.I. (1981) *The Panjabi Language: A Descriptive Grammar. Vol. 2, Languages of Asia and Africa*, Routledge and Kegan Paul, London.

Training in Health and Race (1986a) Communication in health care. *Health and Race*, 3, April, pp. 1–5.

Training in Health and Race (1986b) Improving communication. *Health and Race*, 4, May, pp. 1–5 (Available from Training in Health and Race, 229 Woodhouse Lane, Leeds LS2 9LF.)

Travis, L.E. (ed.) (1971) *Handbook of Speech Pathology and Audiology*, Prentice-Hall, Englewood Cliffs, NJ.

Trudgill, P. (1974) *Sociolinguistics: An Introduction*, Penguin, Harmondsworth.

Volterra, V. and Taeschner, T. (1978) The acquisition and development of language by bilingual children. *Journal of Child Language* 5, 311–26.

Walker, M. (1978) The Makaton Vocabulary. In *Ways and Means* (co-ordinator, T. Tebbs), Globe Education, London.

Walker, M. and Armfield, A. (1981) What is the Makaton Vocabulary? *Special Education: Forward Trends*, **8** (3), 19–20.

Wheldall, K. and Martin, B. (1977) Socio-environmental influences on the receptive language development of young children. *MALS Journal*, **2**, 111–40.

Wheldall, K., Mittler, P. and Hobsbaum, A. (1979) *The Sentence Comprehension Test*, NFER-Nelson, Windsor.

Wheldall, K., Mittler, P., Hobsbaum, A., Duncan, D., Gibbs, D. and Saund, S. (1987) *The Revised Sentence Comprehension Test with the Panjabi Version*, NFER-Nelson, Windsor.

White, L. (1985) The pro-drop parameter in adult second language acquisition. *Language Learning*, **35**, 47–62.

White, L. (1987) Against comprehensible input. *Applied Linguistics*, **8** (2), 95–110.

Wilding, J. (1981) *Ethnic Minority Languages in the Classroom? A Survey of Asian Parents in Leicester*, Leicester Council for Community Relations, Leicester.

Wode, H. (1978) The L1 vs L2 acquisition of English interrogation *Working Papers in Bilingualism*, **15**, 37–58.

Yoshida, M. (1978) The acquisition of English vocabulary by a Japanese-speaking child. In *Second Language Acquisition: A Book of Readings* (ed. E.M. Hatch), Newbury House Publications, Rowley.

Zobl, H. (1980) The formal and developmental selectivity of L1 influence on L2 acquisition. *Language Learning*, **30**, 43–57.

Zobl, H. (1982) A direction for contrastive analysis: the comparative study of developmental sequences. *TESOL Quarterly*, **16** (2) 169–83.

Index